APPEARS
YOUNGER
THAN
STATED
AGE

You've seen the people who always seem young even as they get older. *Now you can be one.*

Doctors have a special designation on patient files: *appears younger than stated age.* What it means is obvious. How you can achieve it is not.

Some people chalk up looking young to good genes. Others to good luck. Dr. Jim Hardeman attributes it to healthy habits. He has developed his approach to looking and feeling younger, healthier, and more vital after years of patient study and personal practice. In clear, everyday language, he details what he's found, including:

- Dietary strategies to preserve the balance of the all-important intake and output of calories
- Fitness habits that will increase your lifespan
- Ways to keep from developing degenerative diseases that so often lead to the vicious cycle of weight gain, inactivity, and deterioration of health
- Simple tips and methods to maintain your ideal body weight

You can begin looking and feeling better at any age. Following Dr. Hardeman's suggestions, you can start dropping years, pounds, and inches and start gaining strength, vitality, and better health.

This is the book that delivers techniques and motivation to transform yourself into someone who looks, feels, and *is* younger than stated age.

APPEARS
YOUNGER
THAN
STATED
AGE

A Doctor's Secrets on the
Art of Staying Young

JAMES L. HARDEMAN, MD

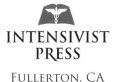

INTENSIVIST
PRESS

FULLERTON, CA

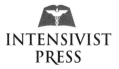
INTENSIVIST PRESS

Intensivist Press
1038 E. Bastanchury Rd. #601
Fullerton, CA 92835

This book shares tools that the author used personally in his quest for well-being, and is intended to educate and entertain. It is not intended to explain, identify or diagnose any condition, medical or otherwise, nor is it intended to replace professional psychological or medical attention, if needed. Although the author and publisher have made every effort to ensure the accuracy and completeness of information contained in this book, we assume no responsibility for errors, inaccuracies, omissions, or any inconsistency herein. The author and publisher shall have neither liability nor responsibility to any person with respect to any loss or damage caused, or alleged to have been caused, directly or indirectly, by the information contained in this book.

Publisher's Cataloging-In-Publication
Hardeman, James L.

   Appears younger than stated age : a doctor's secrets on the art of staying young / James L. Hardeman. -- Fullerton, CA : Intensivist Press, c2012.

   p. ; cm.

   ISBN: 978-0-9857320-1-1; 978-0-9857320-2-8 (trade pbk.); 978-0-9857320-3-5 (ebook)

   Includes bibliographical references and index.

   Summary: Looking young is attributed to healthy habits. Dr. Hardeman's approach to looking and feeling younger, healthier, and more vital is detailed in dietary strategies, fitness habits, tips and methods to maintain ideal body weight, and ways to keep from developing degenerative diseases.--Publisher.

   1. Longevity. 2. Well-being. 3. Vitality. 4. Health. 5. Nutrition. 6. Weight loss. 7. Physical fitness. 8. Aging. 9. Older people--Health and hygiene. 10. Middle-aged persons--Health and hygiene. I. Title. II. Title: Art of staying young.

RA776.75 .H37 2012   2012911174
613/.0434--dc23   1209

Printed in United States of America

Book Consultant: Ellen Reid
Cover Design: Patricia Bacall
Interior Design: Ghislain Viau
Cover & Author photos: Starla Fortunato

This book is gratefully dedicated to my parents for encouraging a strong work ethic, to my children for making me proud, to Kris for everything, and to those who choose to *stay active*.

Table of Contents

Author's Notes

As you read this book, you may notice that the syntax is a little inconsistent. I often use the first person narrative and mix it with other singular and plural pronouns. I am a big proponent of proper grammar and punctuation, but it seemed to make my message too stilted, as did my efforts to present it in the third person. I wanted it to sound as if I'm speaking directly to a patient, and, indeed, much of what I've written in the book has actually been stated to my patients. Therefore, I would like to extend an apology to my influential eleventh grade English teacher, Miss Sandra Beebe, who taught me better than I reveal here.

One of the main themes of this book is ideal body weight maintenance. Although the message is anti-obesity, I would like to make it clear that I am in no way trying to insult obese people. Losing weight is very difficult for many people due to a variety of genetic, social, and psychological influences. Americans collectively agree that we should not discriminate against others on the basis of race, religion, sexual orientation, and disability, and yet scorning the obese seems to be permissible in our contemporary culture. I strongly encourage extending empathy to overweight people and granting them the dignity and respect that everyone deserves. Furthermore, as I explain later, obese patients who exercise and regulate their blood pressure, cholesterol, and glucose levels can actually be healthier than thinner people who do not. And having been left in the dust by many overweight runners in various races, I can guarantee that lanky people are not the only ones who have a fire inside.

Chapter 1

INTRODUCTION

I entered the hospital room and did a double-take. Ada Jones was an eighty-nine-year-old female who needed to see me for a pulmonary consultation because of pneumonia. But this patient did not look eighty-nine. As she rested quietly with eyes closed, I quickly thumbed through her medical record. A phrase caught my eye: "Appears younger than stated age." Evidently I wasn't the only one who had noted her youthful appearance.

I gently woke her and introduced myself, unobtrusively glancing at her hospital identification bracelet to confirm that she was, indeed, Ada Jones. "You look very young for your age," I told her during the course of our conversation. She gave a half-smile and replied, "Well, the pneumonia is sure making me feel older. But soon enough, I'll be back on the tennis court…"

"Appears younger than stated age" is actual medical terminology occasionally placed in the History and Physical (H&P), a document that records an interview and physical exam of every patient admitted to the hospital. Some of the descriptions in the H&P use language that might be undecipherable to non-medical readers. However, general appearance is always commented upon and is more self-explanatory and understandable to all. For example, "alert, awake, and in no acute distress" is a common entry. Although certain factors, such as attractiveness, are not included (one should not compare me to George Clooney on the basis of an H&P, for instance), there is probably no more complimentary a general description than "appears younger than stated age" (AYTSA). The term means what it says: The patient looks good for her age. And it is certainly much better than some of the other terms I've seen and used in an H&P, including: disheveled, disoriented, obese, comatose, or, perhaps worst of all, appears older than stated age.

Why is it then that one ninety-year-old looks seventy-five, lives with his wife self-sufficiently, drives, shops, and even plays a little golf once a week while a seventy-five-year-old looks ninety, resides in a nursing home in a persistent vegetative state, and is fed Ensure through a gastric tube? Or how does one woman at forty-eight have the demeanor of a thirty-five-year-old, run marathons, and ski black diamonds while her younger sister has gained an additional thirty-five pounds, complains of knee pain, has been diagnosed with new-onset diabetes, and could pass for the way older sibling?

Obviously, luck plays a big role in health and often trumps all other factors. Genetics, which falls into the category of luck, is the ultimate uncontrollable aspect of health. Yet there are so many things that we *do* have control over, and AYTSA patients seem to fit a pattern of self-determination, self-discipline, and self-respect.

They are close to their ideal body weights. They don't smoke. They either don't drink alcohol or limit it to one or two drinks per day. They exercise regularly and do not overeat. They seem to be more optimistic than average, and they often are involved in long-term marriages. They take their medications regularly and have periodic checkups. In essence, they are healthy, and healthy people look younger. That's pretty much it. Simple, right? But unfortunately they are more often the exception than the rule.

I can hear the skeptics among you at this juncture. "Sure, simple … in theory." Well, I agree with you … in theory. But the purpose of this book is to demonstrate the relative ease and simplicity of implementing the common-sense principles that will make you look younger and, more importantly, feel younger, whether you are in your twenties or your eighties. And let me be clear that I am not just promoting appearance over substance. We are not talking about the faux youth of plastic surgery or Botox here. People who appear younger than their stated ages are usually *physiologically* younger than their chronologic peers, often simply because they have decided to take better care of themselves. In other words, healthy people not only look younger, but their bodies *function* at a more youthful level,[1] and protective changes may possibly even occur in their bodies' chromosomes as a result of proper diet and exercise.[2] This adds both quantity *and* quality to their lives.

My father was a college history professor, and like most good teachers, he occasionally sprinkled his lectures with life lessons. This analogy is one of my favorites, and I have repeated it countless times to my patients. Imagine that once you learned to drive, you were given a free car of your choosing. But there is a catch: It would be the only car you would own in your entire lifetime. Likely, you would take fanatically good care of your car, washing and waxing it often, changing the oil on schedule, and getting regular maintenance work. Well, this is the only body you'll ever have, so you'd better take very good care of it.

Who is likely to benefit from this book?

- The twenty-year-old who can cement in good health habits that will last a lifetime.
- The thirty-something who is starting to see for the first time the inevitable changes that aging brings.
- The forty-year-old who has been told that life begins in the fifth decade but whose youth seems to be disappearing faster than an object in the rearview.
- The sixty and above crowd who truly can do anything they want if they stay physically fit.

- And, finally, the elderly (whatever age that is) who can participate in more activities and enjoy life to a fuller extent than they ever thought possible.

Although the principles in this book would ideally be started in childhood, people of *any* age can benefit by becoming more fit in both body and mind starting today. There is truly no better time to start than now.

This introduction would not be complete without a more detailed analysis of the expression *appears younger than stated age.* Its origins are unknown. An Internet search reveals very little. A 1993 letter to the editor of *The New England Journal of Medicine* remarks, "An assessment of whether a patient appears younger or older than 'stated age' has long been taught and recorded as a component of the physical exam."[3] The term has been verbally passed from generation to generation of doctors who are particularly suited to make this observation since they are nearly always aware of their patients' ages. My 1976 copy of *DeGowin and DeGowin,*[4] the medical school textbook of how to do a history and physical exam, does not even mention it.

If I were coining the phrase, I might have used "chronologic" instead of "stated" age, because the latter somehow seems to imply that the patient is being less than forthcoming. However, I suspect that the description originated in a simpler time when our culture was less infatuated with youth. It is obviously a subjective assessment, and I am not even certain how relevant it is to the medical record, though the description of the physical exam is intended to convey a medical portrait of the patient—and the phrase certainly does. Regardless of its origins, "appears younger than stated age" is the perfect introduction to a handbook on the art of aging well.

The organization of this book is based upon my approach when discussing medical issues with my patients: identify and describe the problem, understand the causes, and then develop strategies to combat the problem. Although transformation to a healthier lifestyle does not appear as a title until Chapter 5, it is the ultimate theme of this book. To appear younger, to maintain ideal body weight, to live like you mean it, you must transform by adapting the world to you, not the other way around.

The first four chapters of the book deal with identifying and understanding poor health. While this may be a review for some, I have found that many people, even including health care workers, have faulty perceptions due to all the misinformation out there. Subsequently, we will explore the techniques that help to solve the problems. To those who might say, "Yeah, right. Eat less and exercise more; we've heard it all before," the book is really about eating less *indiscriminately* and exercising more *efficiently* and the methods that effectuate these goals.

This is a purposefully slim volume. The chapters are short and the information simple. What I have to impart does not need to be lengthy or complicated. It is a cookbook for good health, concise and with little filler. Critics of the book might suggest that the contents are already so widely known that it's as if I am presenting a treatise on the earth being spherical. Unfortunately, when it comes to responsibility for healthy habits, too many people live in a flat world.

The book was written with the intention that you initially read it cover to cover and refer back to specific chapters later. I have included both advice from my patients and techniques from my own experience, hopefully with enough anecdotes to keep the reader entertained and motivated. Highlighted principles are particularly important, but chapter titles, subheadings used in longer chapters, and the text itself all include essential information. You should be able to finish it in less than a few hours or might feel compelled to read it twice. So what have you got to lose, except the barriers to a healthier and happier you?

Chapter 2

WHY?

"Why do you want to write about diet and health when there are clearly so many other books about the subjects out there?" my wife wondered when I described my book idea. "Furthermore, all the diet books have some gimmick, some magical dietary formula that people think will make them lose weight. They don't want to hear the truth, that eating less and exercising more is the only real way to stay fit."

Well, I guess there are a lot of available books on diet and fitness, and they do have unproven gimmicks from zones to busting sugar to three-week/twenty-pound weight losses to celebrity testimonials. But honestly, though I have leafed through them, I haven't read many from cover to cover because they are too long and boring. Furthermore, I haven't needed them; I have developed my own approach based on scientific research, personal experience, and common sense. And given our increasingly obese and unfit population, *the books that are available are not working.* Why should my book help? Because it is short, succinct, and easy, and although the principles espoused require a lifestyle change, they are certainly not overly burdensome. And I guess that's the gimmick of my book: its brevity and simplicity.

Why should I be the author of such a book? To start with, I have been practicing pulmonary and critical care medicine for more than thirty years and have directly interviewed and examined many thousands of patients. Although I have the utmost respect and admiration for physicians who pursue careers in academic medicine—those who do research and teach at university centers—they usually have a buffer of medical students, interns, and residents between themselves and hands-on care. Yet they are the ones who often write the books. Extensive direct patient care gives me a unique perspective on the requirements for good health.

I have personally questioned hundreds of my patients who have successfully lost weight about their methods. I have seen the adverse health effects of overeating and under-exercising in thousands of patients and have witnessed the perpetual progression of the vicious cycle of poor health. For decades, I have taken an interest in patients who appear younger than their stated ages, and I have listened to what they have told me. Whenever I encounter AYTSA patients, I ask them to reveal the secrets to their youthful appearances. Almost universally, the initial response is that they have tried to stay active for their entire lives. Sometimes their perspectives have been almost startling in their simplicity. One sixty-five-year-old woman with a figure a teenager would envy confided that, to her dismay, her children were starting to gain weight. "They just need some self-discipline," she told me bluntly. "They eat too much."

Furthermore, I avoid hypocrisy in my recommendations to my patients. A healthy diet and regular exercise have been an important part of my life since grade school. I still have my original driver's license from age sixteen, and my weight has remained the same despite college, medical school, residency, a thirty-seven-year marriage, raising two children, and a busy thirty-year medical practice. I know from personal experience how a simple, common sense approach can have a tremendous beneficial impact on one's health and life. My recommendations to my patients are what I say *and* what I do.

Aging gracefully, like medicine itself, is an art based on inexact scientific principles. As I discuss later, we may never be able to do the definitive studies that establish the optimum fitness or weight loss diet. Thus, not all of my statements and recommendations can be backed up with scientific proof, although I have included references when available. I have also relied on personal experience and common sense. Furthermore, even scientific dogma is relative. What was thought to be factual yesterday may be disproved today and vice versa.

When faced with any medical dilemma, the all-important question you should ask your physician is, "If it were you, what would you do?" Since much of this book revolves around my own methods developed through trial and error and later passed on to my patients, I often discuss my personal experiences with regard to health and fitness. I do not mean to be boastful. On the contrary, apart from my lifelong effort to stay physically fit, I am very ordinary. Never a gifted athlete, I am neither strong nor fast, and I have been only average in my sporting endeavors. As a member of the middle of the bell curve, I believe that what has worked for me can work for you. I am just like you, and I take care of patients just like all of us; if we can do it, so can you.

Chapter 3

HIGH SCHOOL REUNION

(OBESITY IN AMERICA)

There are few events in one's life where appearance is more emphasized than at high school reunions. There you are, drink in hand, adorned with a nametag and photograph of your eighteen-year-old self when you were likely at your physical prime, wondering if your former classmates will recognize or remember you.

Having been to my tenth, twentieth, and thirtieth high school reunions, I have discerned a not so subtle trend: although the yearbook photos remain static, the majority of my previous fellow students have become almost unrecognizable because of progressive weight gain, and this most certainly does not make them appear younger. Year after year at countless high school reunions throughout the country, the same scenario plays out.

A stroll through nearly any mall in America will confirm that we have become a nation with an obesity problem. Sixty-seven percent of us are overweight and thirty-four percent are actually obese.[1] One of the world's cruelest ironies is that certain populations are still starving to death while others, like our own, are dying prematurely because of too much food. And startling statistics don't seem to faze us; less than ten percent of a recent study population embraced a healthy lifestyle.[2]

How and why did we get to this point?

I believe the most important factor in our growing obesity problem is that evolution never intended for us to count calories or limit our food intake. In fact, we are genetically designed to stuff ourselves … and to stuff ourselves with calorically dense fuel (i.e., fat) and brain food (i.e., sugar, the energy substrate of the brain).[3] Indeed, had our ancestors not gorged themselves at times when food was plentiful, they would not have built up the fat stores necessary for survival during leaner times, and likely none of us would even be here.

Furthermore, it seems that eating begets more eating, probably another genetic adaptation to encourage us to eat as much as possible when food is available. Who has not experienced the difficulty in eating just one potato chip or just one chocolate? Rather than partially satiate us, it simply creates a craving for more. It is easier to resist the temptation of the first bite of food than it is to stop once we've started to eat.

Evolution apparently never anticipated easy access to food. First of all, nutritional deficiencies and infectious diseases limited life expectancy in the past such that people generally did not live long enough to develop obesity and its attendant complications. Life was "nasty, brutish and short" in the words of seventeenth-century English philosopher Thomas Hobbes, and simply making it to reproductive age and procreating was the genetic bottom line.

Furthermore, food had to be chased, hunted, picked, or cultivated, requiring much more caloric expenditure than the modern day equivalent: walking to the refrigerator for a second bowl of ice cream. Contemporary society enjoys the luxury of very accessible, great-tasting food along with effort-saving devices that decrease the need for activity—an ideal recipe for developing obesity and its consequences.

While reigning in our appetites might seem to be a hopeless endeavor given our evolutionary predisposition to overeat, we likewise have been genetically blessed with human traits such as reason, free will, and self-discipline that help us to resist the tendency to eat too much. It is important to understand what we are up against but also to recognize that we possess the tools to conquer it. This brings us to the first principle in this book.

PRINCIPLE 1

Pursuit of a healthy lifestyle
requires a personal transformation.

For a lucky few, their goals, values, likes, and dislikes coincide with those of a healthy lifestyle, but for many, if not most, people, this process requires a change. Immediate gratification, particularly poor dietary and exercise habits, must be replaced by something more long lasting and substantive. We must change our attitudes on life and not allow food to control us. Our natural tendency toward inertia needs to yield to activity. And what is always a lifelong pursuit, the search for self identity,[4] needs to be channeled into a better looking and better feeling you. You will reach a point where a fit, healthy person is not just what you are; it is who you are. The time to change is now. How to change is what this book is all about.

So … when you attend your next high school reunion, and you bump into the ex-jock whose eyes move from your face to your nametag and back to your face, he just might say, without a trace of the irony that he may have used years ago, "Wow, you look really good." You can humbly reply, "Thank you," but inside, you'll be saying to yourself, *I know.*

Chapter 4

ZPG

ZERO POPULATION GROWTH
FOR YOUR FAT CELLS

It has only been during a recent tiny segment on the time line of humanity beginning with the industrial revolution a few hundred years ago that a dissociation between food availability and survival has occurred in certain populations. In the United States, relatively inexpensive high quality nutrition can be obtained by nearly everyone. In fact, too much food is available too easily; it often tastes too temptingly good, and it is too calorically dense, that is, high in calories for its weight. Consequently, maintaining one's ideal body weight has become increasingly difficult in our modern society.

Ideal Body Weight (IBW) is basically what you should weigh for your height, gender, and frame size. There is no greater factor in looking, feeling, and being younger than your stated age than maintaining your ideal body weight for your entire life. And almost nothing will make you look older than a panniculus of belly fat hanging over your belt or the buttery jowls of a double chin that quiver as you speak. IBW connotes youth, vitality, and a sense of self-respect. The main focus of this book is to convince you to maintain IBW. If you're there, stay there. If you're not, get there, and never leave.

How Much Should I Weigh?

Ideal body weight information is based on actuarial data from insurance companies and determinations of body fat percentages in large populations. A number of formulas for IBW can be found on the Internet, but here is an easy one:

Males: 106 pounds + 6 x inches over 5 feet

Females: 100 pounds + 5 x inches over 5 feet

Then determine frame size as follows: grasp your wrist with your thumb and index finger. If they just touch, you have a medium-sized frame and no adjustment is needed. If there is a gap, you have a large frame and add 10% to the above formula. And if they overlap as far as the fingernail bed, you are small framed, and subtract 10%.[1] For example, a 5' 4" medium-frame woman's IBW would be 100 (pounds) + 5 x 4 (inches over 5 feet) = 120 pounds.

Another parameter to determine proper weight is the body mass index, or BMI—again an assessment of weight in relationship to height. In scientific literature, BMI has largely replaced IBW as the method of choice to document and follow an individual's appropriate weight. However, weight in pounds is a simpler number to which most people can more easily relate. Therefore, throughout this book, the term IBW is utilized, but "normal BMI" could be used interchangeably. You can determine your BMI by referring to tables readily available on the Internet or by utilizing the following method:

Weight in pounds x 703 = X

X ÷ height in inches = Y

Y ÷ height in inches = BMI

Ideal body weight generally correlates with a BMI of less than 25. A higher BMI is usually due to the accumulation of too much fat tissue or, in scientific terminology, adipose tissue. A BMI of 25 to

30 is considered overweight, of 30 to 40, obese, and over 40 earns the distinctly unpleasant designation of morbid obesity. Caveats in interpretation should be considered in very lean, muscular individuals, short women (five feet or below), and those who are pregnant, all of whom may have high BMI without actually having excessive adipose tissue.[2] For our 5' 4"/120-pound woman, BMI would be 120 (pounds) x 703 = 84360. 84360 ÷ 64 (inches) = 1318 ÷ 64 (inches) = 20.6, well within the normal BMI range.

A third method to assess proper weight is waist circumference, which tells more about the distribution of fat than the percentage of total body fat. The importance of body fat and the value of real estate may have something in common: location, location, location. People who accumulate fat in the abdomen (apple shape) tend to have a greater incidence of high blood pressure, elevated cholesterol, diabetes, and heart disease than those who have fat buttocks and thighs (pear shape). The reasons for this divergence are not entirely clear, but abdominal fat acts differently than that in other locations, possibly releasing chemical compounds that are deleterious to health.[3]

To measure waist size, stand up, and use a tape measure. Place it at the point below your rib cage but above the top of the pelvic bone (iliac crests) with your breath normally (not forcefully) exhaled. The tape will usually be a little above the navel.[4] If your BMI is more than 30, don't bother with this measurement because you are already at risk for disease because of your weight. If your BMI is less than 30, a waist size more than thirty-five inches for a woman or forty inches for a man puts you at higher risk as well.[5]

WHAT IS A CALORIE?

A calorie is the unit used to designate the energy value of food, or, if not used immediately for energy, the food's weight gain potential. Technically, it is the amount of heat required to raise the temperature of one gram of water at sea level by one degree Celsius.[6] When referring to food, one calorie is actually so tiny that it needs to be multiplied by 1000 to be significant, and, therefore, the real name is kilocalorie. By convention, however, everyone nowadays simply calls a kilocalorie a calorie.[7] When you eat food with lots of calories, some will be used for energy immediately, but any leftover calories can be converted to fat and stored in the body for future use if necessary. Hence, the more calories you eat, the more likely you are to gain weight in the form of fat.

Calories are also a measure of how much energy a certain activity requires. More intense activities produce higher caloric requirements. Thus, the energy expenditure of standing for thirty minutes is 44 calories; of walking (3 mph), 120 calories; and of running (5.2 mph), 330 calories.[8] Simply stated, the more active you are, the less prone you will be to weight gain. As we will discuss in more detail later, one pound of body fat is worth about 3500 calories.[9]

INTAKE AND OUTPUT (I&O)

A stroll down the aisle of the diet and health section of almost any bookstore reveals a plethora of books by a diverse cross-section of humanity: MDs, PhDs, celebrities, dietitians, firemen, French women, and other self-styled gurus. Most of them promote mystical dietary formulas: low and high carbohydrate, no sugar, low and high fat, "magic" foods, diets based on blood type—the list goes on and on. What they don't say is that there is no scientific evidence that one weight loss diet is better than another as long as it restricts caloric intake.[10]

And this brings us to the universal truth about weight loss and maintenance, which is expressed in one simple concept: the balance of intake and output of calories, I&O. Though admittedly somewhat more difficult in practice than theory, there is no question that altering the balance of food intake (I) and energy expenditure or output (O) can markedly affect your weight.

PRINCIPLE 2

It's all I&O, intake and output of calories.

I&O is why the Atkins Diet, the South Beach Diet, the Sugar Busters Diet, and all the rest can be effective because *they limit the intake of calories.* If your intake of calories is approximately the same as output, your weight will remain about the same. This is what you want to do if you are already at your IBW. If you increase your food intake but keep exercise the same, you'll gain weight. And you can lose weight by decreasing how much you eat (I) or increasing your activity level (O) or both. It's as simple as that.

I believe that the MyPlate guidelines, promoted by the USDA and the Department of Health and Human Services (see Chapter 9), are as close to the gold standard of good nutrition as it gets. Many fad diets, however, claim that, by adjusting nutritional components of the diet, one can more easily lose weight. The three main nutritional components of food, called macronutrients, are protein, fat, and carbohydrate. Fat is more calorically dense with 9 calories per gram while protein and carbohydrate are about half that with 4 calories per gram each. That means you can eat twice as much carbohydrate by weight as fat for the same number of calories, a fact that gives credence to the concept of low fat diets for weight reduction. I should mention, however, that fat in the stomach may delay gastric emptying,[11] thereby diminishing hunger and curbing appetite in a calorically restricted weight reduction diet.

THE *NEW ENGLAND JOURNAL* STUDY

The best and most recent study of dietary components comes from the most prestigious medical journal in the world, the *New England Journal of Medicine*, in February 2009. Researchers from

Harvard and other university centers divided 800 overweight or obese subjects into four groups based on diets that differed in percentages of the macronutrients: carbohydrate, fat, and protein. The two-year study included group sessions and biochemical monitoring to ensure compliance with the diets. Results showed that weight loss occurred from a calorie-restricted diet *without regard* to differing percentages of fat, carbohydrate, and protein. Interestingly, fullness, hunger, and satisfaction with the diets were similar for all groups. Their conclusion was that total calorie intake was the determining factor in weight loss, not the components of the diet.[12]

However ... there are some problems with the study. Although long for a study of its type, it only lasted for two years, not a lifetime of IBW maintenance that I'm promoting. Subjects only lost an average of four kilograms or about nine pounds. They only exercised moderately for ninety minutes per week, far less than I would recommend for weight maintenance, let alone weight loss. The diets were designed to be similar but did not look and taste exactly the same. Biochemical tests suggested that not all participants adhered completely to their prescribed diets.

An editorial comment about the article in the same issue of the *New England Journal* opined that the only way to be certain as to their conclusions would be to make the four diets look and taste the same. To do this might require porridges with different components of carbohydrates, protein, and fat, and it is unlikely that study volunteers would agree to eating gruel three meals a day for the several years it would take to complete the experiment. Thus, a definitive study to assess dietary components may never be done.[13] In the meantime, this article is probably the best proof yet that the I&O principle reigns supreme.

To further illustrate, let us take extreme examples of I&O. Famine will prevent obesity in everyone, even those with the greatest genetic predisposition to being overweight.[14] Likewise, if you were able to run a marathon every day, it is very unlikely that obesity would be a problem for you. Obviously, neither of these methods is a realistic solution to the problem of weight maintenance, but the principle stands: we need to restrict our food intake enough and exercise enough to maintain our ideal body weights. The purpose of this book is to demonstrate just how easy and practical these methods can be. But first, let us discuss some of the complexities of both intake and output of calories.

INTAKE

Food intake is controlled by brain signals and hormone influence, and both hereditary and environmental factors may affect appetite. We surmise that hunger is what causes us to eat. However, even morbidly obese people, who could live for months without food, experience hunger. And who among us has not felt satiated by a meal only to eat more when the sight or smell of a tempting food entices us? Appetite is influenced by sight, smell, intestinal distension, and hormones, in addition to cultural and psychological factors.[15]

There actually does exist a weak feedback mechanism whereby a hormone—leptin, secreted by fat cells—decreases appetite and increases energy expenditure. The more fat cells, the more leptin. Unfortunately, certain obese people may have leptin resistance where the part of the brain that controls appetite, the hypothalamus, does not respond normally to leptin.[16] Much research is ongoing, and eventually a safe appetite-suppressing drug or hormone will be developed and perhaps render much of this book obsolete.

It might seem that there is so much biological propensity to overeat—and such an abundance of good-tasting food in our modern world—that maintaining ideal body weight is simply a losing battle. On the other hand, as I will state repeatedly in this book, we are not wild animals or cavemen. We are capable of applying reason and self-discipline to most aspects of our lives, including diet. And as opposed to our ancestors who ate hand to mouth, we can be fairly certain that our next meal is not in jeopardy.

OUTPUT

Caloric output, energy expenditure, the burning of calories, or whatever you want to call it, is a little more interesting than intake because so much of it occurs without our having to do anything at all. Energy expenditure can be roughly divided into physical activity, approximately 10%, and basal metabolic rate, approximately 70%. The remainder is due to other mechanisms such as the energy-burning requirement of metabolizing food.[17] Basal metabolic rate, BMR, is the energy we utilize from just being alive. You might simply be sitting on the couch reading this, but, even at rest, your cells are working like crazy. It is fascinating that we burn more than two thirds of our calories without even lifting a finger. However … the rules change as we get older.

When we are young, BMR is like a raging furnace that allows us to eat almost anything and not seem to gain weight. Sadly, however, BMR decreases by about 2 to 3% every decade past age twenty-five.[18] Part of the reason is that as people age, they have less muscle mass and more fat, and muscle metabolism burns more calories than does fat.[19] So, when a patient comes to the office stating that he's gaining weight even though his food intake and activity level have been the same for the past twenty years, there is a reason for that. Although not proven, I suspect that we probably burn calories with exercise less efficiently as we grow older, as well. Thus, many people in their thirties and forties reach what has been called "metabolic menopause," whereby the intake and output balance becomes increasingly unfavorable. As the years go by, you simply must eat a little less and exercise a little more if you want to maintain your ideal body weight.

Some of you might wonder at this point why our metabolic rates decrease with age. What evolutionary advantage might this have conferred? We'll never know for sure, but one can theorize. As humans age they quickly leave the peak of their physical prowess; naturally, our older ancestors would have been less adept at hunting/gathering than their younger counterparts. A decreased BMR would mean a little lower requirement for obtaining food. Alternatively, perhaps a lower BMR improves survival by allowing the cells to last longer. In either case, those with decreased BMRs could have lived longer, reproduced more often, and therefore have had a genetic advantage. (Feel free to ponder other theories on your own, but take a walk while you do so, won't you?)

As with the case of intake of food, output of calories is complicated by the effects of modern society. Our ancestors were forced to be active, but nowadays there are so many physical energy-saving devices that a sedentary lifestyle is not only possible but common. Again, self-discipline allows us to compensate by increasing our levels of physical exercise.

OBESITY

Obesity is basically a defense mechanism against starving. We can store energy in fat cells, or adipocytes, for later so that we can live for up to several months without starving to death.[20] Adipocytes store fat in the form of triglycerides that can later be broken down to free fatty acids which are used by other body cells for energy. When we lose weight, we are basically using fat deposits of previously ingested food, or, as one of my friends from medical school used to claim when he skipped a meal, "I'm eating fat for lunch."

It is not necessary to consume actual fat in the diet to become overweight as there are also metabolic pathways in the body to convert excess amounts of dietary carbohydrates and protein to triglyceride for storage in adipocytes.[21] As we have discussed, however, dietary fat is twice as calorically dense as protein or carbohydrates, so it is easier to take on excessive calories when consuming foods high in fat.

Controversy exists as to cell number versus cell size in adipose tissue. In scientific terms, *hyperplasia* means new fat cells are created while *hypertrophy* refers to more fat contained per fat cell. It used to be thought that only children and adolescents could develop new fat cells, but this may also occur in adults.[22] Common sense might indicate that the existence of more fat cells might make weight loss more difficult and perhaps have significant implications for childhood obesity, i.e., overweight children who develop more fat cells could be facing more difficult obesity problems as adults. A recent University of Iowa study may support this contention. Five-year-olds who were more active than their counterparts weighed less than their peers when they reached age eleven whether their activity levels persisted or not.[23] These theories are not proven but emphasize the advice, "Start early, but it is never too late to adopt a healthy lifestyle."

ADVERSE CONSEQUENCES OF OBESITY

Obesity is a lethal disease; obese people have a 50-100% increased risk of dying prematurely. It is the second leading cause of preventable death in the United States. (If you can't guess what the first is, see Chapter 11.)

Specific conditions associated with obesity include:

a. Cardiovascular disease—hypertension (high blood pressure), heart attacks, and heart failure.

b. Cerebrovascular disease—strokes and some types of dementia.

c. Diabetes mellitus—elevated glucose (blood sugar) which is associated with premature artery disease and often leads to heart, kidney, eye, nerve, and brain diseases.

d. Certain types of cancer including colon, breast, pancreas, prostate, uterus, and ovary.

e. Hyperlipidemia (high cholesterol), which increases the incidence of strokes and heart attacks.

f. Sleep apnea—intermittent pauses in breathing while asleep. Sleep apnea can lead to profound tiredness, psychological changes, and heart problems.

g. GERD—gastroesophageal reflux disease or heartburn.

h. Arthritis—due to increased weight burden on joints, especially knees and hips.

i. Gallstones.

j. Loss of self-esteem.[24]

k. Adipose tissue may turn out to be the largest endocrine, i.e., hormone-producing, organ in the body with as yet undetermined adverse effects.[25]

INTAKE, OUTPUT, AND OBESITY

One big problem with weight gain is that it is not at all an immediate occurrence. We don't wake up the morning after having eaten a large dinner to find we have gained five pounds. Instead, it is an insidious process, much the same way high cholesterol causes artery narrowing by gradually, over the years, creating plaque. We don't perceive the immediate effects of second helpings or rich desserts, but with enough time they become obvious. Even small alterations of I&O balance can have profound implications. A 1% positive imbalance of intake over output for thirty years could lead to a weight gain of sixty pounds![26]

PRINCIPLE 3

*People tend to overestimate output
and underestimate intake.*

Therefore, it is important to keep track of intake and output of calories and weigh yourself daily. Men need to eat about 11 calories per pound of weight; and females, 10 for basic metabolic needs. The gender difference is explained by the fact that males have less fat and more muscle than females, and muscle metabolism burns more calories than does fat. Thus, a 150-pound man would require a minimum of 1650 calories. Taking activity into consideration, however, multiply weight in pounds by 13 for low activity and by 15 for moderate activity.[27] Thus, our 150-pound man might require as much as 2250 calories for total energy expenditure.

Another way of estimating calorie requirements is by means of age and activity level, as shown in the table below. Since basal metabolic rate begins to decrease after about age twenty-five, age adjustment is necessary. Several other much more complicated equations exist for calorie requirement estimation, but they have limited utility when dealing with the goal of ideal body weight maintenance. If you are already maintaining your IBW, general awareness of caloric intake is still prudent, though closely counting calories is not really necessary. And if you do start gaining weight, the only calories you need to count are the ones by which you are decreasing your input and/or those by which you are increasing your output.

Gender	Age (years)	Sedentary	Moderately Active	Active
Female	19-30	2,000	2,000-2,200	2,400
	31-50	1,800	2,000	2,200
	51+	1,600	1,800	2,000-2,200
Male	19-30	2,400	2,600-2,800	3,000
	31-50	2,200	2,400-2,600	2,800-3,000
	51+	2,000	2,200-2,400	2,400-2,800

Sedentary indicates only light physical activity that would occur in usual activities of daily living.

Moderately active indicates physical activity equivalent to walking 1.5 to 3 miles per day at 3 to 4 mph plus activities of daily living.

Active indicates physical activity equivalent to walking more than 3 miles per day at 3 to 4 mph plus activities of daily living.

Adapted from Dietary Guidelines for Americans, 2005, www.hhs.gov

It is useful to equate food calories with expenditure calories. I&O can easily get out of balance if we use indiscretion in food intake as illustrated in what I call the Milky Way®-Mile Principle: eat a Milky Way, walk a mile. At Halloween, smaller versions of candy bars are often given to trick-or-treaters, including a Milky Way Fun Bar, which measures about 2x1 inches and is one-half inch thick. It is easy to eat two or three of these at one sitting, and, amazingly, each one is packed with 80 calories. Walking a mile leads to the burning of approximately 80 calories and certainly requires far more time and effort than eating one little Milky Way. Just think how far you would have to walk to make up for a jumbo-sized candy bar! This type of risk-reward assessment is a useful endeavor when confronted with the temptation to eat some treat for immediate gratification rather than to actually alleviate hunger. It also emphasizes the importance of reading nutrition labels and counting calories. Remember that one pound of fat represents 3500 calories. And 3500 calories is the equivalent of eating seven Big Macs® (intake) or running thirty-five miles (output.)

Obesity is a vicious cycle disease. Weight gain leads to health problems and less ability to exercise which, in turn, causes more obesity, making exercise even more difficult, and on and on. Maintaining your ideal body weight is much easier than getting it back once your weight has become out of control ... which leads to the next principle.

PRINCIPLE 4

If your weight goes above 5% over your ideal body weight, do something now.

Referring back to our 150-pound man, a 5% gain would be 150 x .05 = 7.5 pounds. At this point he must go into full-fledged weight loss mode using the advice in Chapter 16 until he is back to his ideal body weight. It is much more difficult and frustrating to get back to your IBW if you have added an extra twenty or thirty pounds than it is to maintain within 5% of a lean version of yourself.

I am a little reluctant to write this next paragraph because I do not want to discourage anyone from getting to their IBW. But what should you do if you've tried and tried and simply can't? First of all, never stop trying, because evidence shows that people who have attempted weight loss many times before can eventually be successful.[28] In the meantime, rather than despair, I would encourage you to be as healthy as you can within that context. You should still follow the advice of this book, and even small amounts of weight loss can often ameliorate some of the adverse consequences of obesity. Furthermore, pharmacologic control of blood pressure, diabetes, and cholesterol, along with regular exercise and sensible food consumption, can render even an obese person relatively healthy.

Summary

The importance of this chapter cannot be overemphasized and warrants recapitulation. Maintaining ideal body weight is the *sine qua non* of twenty-first century health, and it is all based on the intake and output of calories. Our evolutionary genetic tendency toward overeating—plus the conveniences and abundant food of our modern times—have combined to form the perfect storm for an obesity epidemic. Our genetic makeup, however, also includes strength of conviction and willpower to combat this tempest. This section has presented the essential concepts, but it is in future chapters that you'll see how straightforward the practical applications of healthy living can be.

Chapter 5

TRANSFORMATION

U p until this point we have discussed health and fitness theory more than practicality. We can understand why there is a tendency for people to become overweight in modern society. The intake and output principle is the generality, but now we will begin to explore the specifics of weight maintenance.

The next two chapters, *Workout* and *Bring Your Lunch*, may provoke skepticism because they will promote more exercise and more dietary alteration than you might have imagined. I am asking you not to toss the book aside in disbelief but to carefully read it and consider embracing a lifestyle that you will never regret.

Our ancestors expended whatever energy was necessary to obtain food and ate whatever was available to survive, whether it was reptiles, rodents, insects … and probably even each other. Monotonous meals were likely commonplace. Picky eaters didn't live long. Humans only relatively recently have been able to choose from an array of foods, but our very existence is proof that we can thrive on what may not be our first food choices for immediate gratification. So when people say they just can't exercise more or can't abandon their meat and potatoes mindset, they really mean that they *won't*.

In modern society, the temptation to overeat and the tendency toward being inactive are battles we never seem to win because they are easier than the alternatives, not because they make us feel better in the long run. Life is obviously a series of trade-offs. Some people believe that inactivity, a saturated fat laden diet, and obesity are preferable to a less hedonistic lifestyle, even if it means a shorter life span. At least that's what they think when they're younger. From talking with hundreds of patients in poor health in their sixties and seventies, however, I know that many wish they would have shown a little more dietary restraint and exercise motivation in years past.

Research increasingly indicates that living a healthy lifestyle has tremendous benefits, and the transformation doesn't even need to be complicated. A recent University of Cambridge study showed that participants who didn't smoke, were physically active, ate five servings of fruits or vegetables daily, and limited alcohol intake would live fourteen years longer than those who did not.[1] Another study, entitled "Healthy Living Is the Best Revenge," demonstrated that people could be 80% healthier by doing only four things: exercising regularly, avoiding obesity (body mass index less than 30), never smoking, and eating a healthy diet (fruits, vegetables, whole grains, and little meat). Shockingly, only 9% of the 23,153 subjects in the latter study adhered to all four of these factors![2]

For the sake of example, I have included specific details of my daily intake and output of calories. I am quite certain that if you are at your IBW, and if you eat and exercise as I do, then you will maintain your ideal weight. But what I really want is for you to use my recommendations as a template. I hope that you develop your own diet, workout regimen, and enhanced activities of daily living based on your own interests and food preferences. Help in this endeavor can be found on a number of websites including calorieking.com, eatright.org, and choosemyplate.gov.

This book is all about convincing you to adopt the AYTSA lifestyle, and once you are at ideal body weight and perhaps in the best shape of your life, the success will be self-perpetuating and self-reinforcing.

Healthy living envelops us 24/7, while eating a few donuts or taking a nap is so transient.

So read on with an open mind. Don't slam the book closed and say you can't do it. Try to embrace the transformation, and discover that the journey of fitness and healthy eating is itself the reward.

Chapter 6

WORKOUT

The clock radio alarm goes off early in my household, almost always before there is even a hint of light sky in the sky. And nearly every morning I lie torpid in bed for several minutes before finally convincing myself to get up and start working out. How is it, I often ask myself, that someone as dedicated to exercise as I still must force himself to start? Why is something that makes us feel so alive and so good about ourselves so difficult to initiate? The moment of truth, that time between lying comfortably in a warm bed and pounding the pavement, is often the only thing that separates an AYTSA person from the rest. And even ten steps into my run, I'm already glad that I opted for another morning workout.

PRINCIPLE 5

You must will yourself to overcome the moment of truth.

The psychological barrier to initiate a workout is common and may, obviously, thwart a daily exercise regimen. One wonders if our forebears felt this way before embarking upon the hunt or rising to tend the crops, or did nutritional necessity motivate them to immediately spring into action? Modern day exercise is basically a simulation of the physical activity that was forced upon our ancestors, and perhaps our minds reason that it is not the prerequisite for survival that it once was. Yet, in an inverted way, it is still necessary for long-term survival.

THE BENEFITS OF EXERCISE

The advantages of regular exercise are legion. *Harrison's Principles of Internal Medicine* lists in the index no fewer than nineteen conditions for which exercise is recommended, from cardiac disease to osteoporosis to fibromyalgia. Regular exercise lowers blood pressure, decreases cholesterol, and keeps glucose better controlled in diabetics.[1] It is a great stress reliever and is often recommended as a nonpharmacologic treatment for anxiety and depression.[2] Furthermore, it may actually diminish the likelihood of developing dementia later in life.[3]

BORN TO RUN

Humans were designed to exercise. Observation of any school playground confirms that exercise is an innate human characteristic. Indeed, had our ancestors not been able to walk, run, lift, throw, push, pull, and climb we would not likely be here today. There were no such things as cave potatoes. Exercise should be a part of everyone's daily routine from the cradle to the grave, just as eating, sleeping, and brushing teeth are. We generally do not consider that brushing our teeth three times a week is sufficient, and exercise should be looked at in the same manner.

PRINCIPLE 6

Exercise every day.

Recommendations in the past have encouraged participation in moderate exercise three to four times a week. This might be sufficient if you are in your mid-twenties, but remember that basal metabolic rate decreases by 2 to 3% each decade after age twenty-five.[4] Thus, increasing your exercise regimen with age makes sense if you want to preserve caloric intake and output balance. Furthermore, recent evidence from the National Weight Control Registry has shown that people who have lost significant weight and kept it off exercise an average of sixty to ninety minutes daily,[5] far more than was traditionally thought necessary. I recommend a regimen that combines walking or running one day with weight lifting the next. This provides for the expenditure of calories in addition to the development of muscle mass. Again, more muscle helps to perpetuate weight maintenance since muscle metabolism burns more calories than fat. In fact, muscle metabolism can be responsible for 20% of basal metabolic rate, and trained, muscular athletes can actually have a 5% greater BMR just from increased muscle mass.[6] This is like burning calories for free! It is important to note studies have not proven that the combination of weight lifting and aerobics (running or walking) is superior to either activity alone with respect to weight loss, however.[7]

Of course, the everyday workout should be only a part of your caloric expenditure since activities of daily living and recreational pursuits burn calories as well (see Chapter 13, *Take the Stairs*). However, a dedicated daily workout is an essential part of transformation to a healthy lifestyle.

GET IT DONE EARLY

The timing of exercise is optional, though I am a strong proponent of doing it early in the morning before work. Like a financial planner's concept of saving 10% of each paycheck before you spend on anything else, you are paying yourself first with fitness and good health. Bad days and late evenings at work have a way of destroying motivation, and having already done it in the morning gives you the peace of mind that you've already fit exercise into your schedule. And this may sound like heresy to some of you, but even on weekends or days off, getting up early to exercise is advisable. Adopt a workout routine and adhere to it until it becomes a part of you. There are, of course, many people who prefer to exercise after their workday. Pragmatism rules, and you should adhere to whatever functions for you as long as it can be sustained for a lifetime.

WALKING AND RUNNING

In my college physics class, the professor asked for two volunteers, one to walk and one to run up the stairs of the auditorium. *Which student burned more calories?* the professor wanted to know. His surprising answer: they expended the same amount. Newton's laws of motion dictated that the energy used to move mass (the students' bodies) over distance (the stairs) was independent of the speed with which it was done. For years the concept that both running and walking a mile burned 100 calories was accepted as common knowledge. The only difference was how long it took. After all, who was going to argue with Sir Isaac Newton?

However … recent studies confirm that while Newton was right, the physics professor was not. In 2004, Syracuse University researchers used sophisticated methods to measure calorie expenditure in subjects who ran and walked 1600 meters (about a mile). Men burned 124 calories running and 88 walking, while women expended 105 and 74, respectively, for the same activities. People who weigh more expend more calories per activity, which accounts for the gender difference.

So how do Newton's motion laws explain this? Probably because running involves a jumping motion as one moves from foot to foot, and thus additional work is done against gravity as compared to the rather straight leg configuration of walking.

Even more difference was found when the *net calorie burn* (NCB) was taken into account. NCB is the difference between total calories burned and those attributed to basal metabolic rate, which, you will remember, is the number of calories the runners would have burned had they spent that time simply sitting on the couch doing nothing. For men, NCB running was 105 calories and walking, 52; and in women, 91 and 43, respectively.[8]

Both running and walking are excellent exercises, and they are unique in that they are innate. Most other activities, such as swimming or riding a bicycle, require skills that are learned, while running and walking just happen. The difference in calories expended between walking and running, however, has profound implications when applied to the intake and output principle. You will have to spend more time and go farther to walk off the same number of calories that you would burn running.

In Defense of Walking

Although runners may tend to regard walking as a wimpy exercise, nothing could be further from the truth.[9] For most people, walking is likely to form the foundation of their calorie expending activities, and it is certainly effective. One study demonstrated that Amish subjects took six times as many daily steps as average American adults and, despite diets that were not very healthy, had a nearly 90% lower incidence of obesity.[10] Walking can be done any time, in nearly any weather, either alone or with friends. It is not uncomfortable, rarely leads to injuries, and is conducive to carrying on a conversation with a walking partner. While running is a more concentrated calorie-burning endeavor, adjustments in your walking distance can result in the same caloric expenditure as running. And even runners will find that supplemental walking can help maintain a favorable intake and output balance.

Specific Workout

Much of this book is intended to be specific, so I will describe in detail the workout to which I adhere. Obviously, it will need to be individualized. You will need to start slowly and then progressively increase the regimen until goal activity is achieved, probably over a period of months. And if you are over age forty or fifty with a family history of heart disease, get a clearance from your physician before you start.

a. Run or walk 4.5 miles Tuesday, Thursday, and Sunday. Remember that you will need to walk farther than you might run in order to burn the same number of calories.

b. Lift weights Monday, Wednesday, Friday, and Saturday, including bench presses, curls, reverse curls, one-armed curls, chest hoists, side lifts, and behind the head lifts. This regimen should take about 45 minutes and is further delineated in the Appendix. Weight lifting not only burns calories and increases muscle mass, but also strengthens muscles that can protect joints and keep you safer during recreational endeavors. My preference is to use free weights because of convenience and low expense, but admittedly a universal machine at home (if you can afford it) or at the gym may be safer and eliminates the possibility of dropping something on your foot.

c. Daily calisthenics including push-ups (40), pull-ups (14), and sit-ups or abdominal crunches (150). For women, push-ups on palms and knees are acceptable, and pull-ups may need to be simulated with gym equipment.

d. Engage in exercise-related hobbies several times per week. Not only can they consume calories and promote a better sense of balance, they are also fun. Inert hobbies can be transformed into active ones including hiking, bicycling, rollerblading, golfing (walking the course), playing tennis or racquetball, skiing, snowboarding, surfing or boogie boarding, and gardening. The daily workout becomes complementary to such activities since it keeps you always prepared to enjoy these fun, more intermittent recreational pursuits. One note of caution: if you engage in gravity or acceleration-related sports, don't ever neglect to protect your melon with a good quality helmet.

The above workout, along with the activities of daily living (see Chapter 6, *Take the Stairs*) and calorie-burning hobbies will provide an average of 1½ to 2 hours of exercise per day, an amount that I consider essential to weight maintenance and good health. Two hours initially sounds like a daunting amount of exercise, but remember that only about half of it actually represents a dedicated workout. Furthermore, we are transforming ourselves from a mindset that exercise is a chore to one where it is a hobby. Exercise becomes a means of self-identification, and it is as much a part of us as our professions and families.

PRACTICALITY

Once a vow has been made for daily exercise, however, the major challenge is to maintain it over years, over decades, over a lifetime. And this brings us to the next principle.

PRINCIPLE 7

Keep it simple and keep it comfortable.

The more simple a workout, the more likely that it will not be abandoned. That is why I favor having equipment at home rather going to a gym, travel to which involves one more intermediary step toward a workout. The gym obviously functions for many people as a motivating factor. Exercise partners are more available and certainly gym equipment is better than my meager home setup. So if a gym keeps you exercising daily, go with it.

For many people like me, however, exercise in solitude is preferable. I am not very muscular or strong and feel a little self-conscious pumping iron in front of others. Furthermore, less motivation is required to roll out of bed and start my workout than to drive to the gym before starting. Certainly home equipment saves time and, after all, isn't *I just haven't had the time* the most common excuse for not exercising? Studies actually suggest that home equipment may enhance exercise compliance and weight maintenance.[11]

My plain vanilla home gym consists of a weight bench, a universal bar, curling bars, dumbbells, a pull-up bar, and the streets of my neighborhood. If I lived in a cold or rainy climate I would definitely also have a treadmill and a stationary bicycle. While not inexpensive, these items are within most people's budgets and will eventually be cheaper than year after year of a gym membership and certainly much less expensive than the illnesses they may help prevent.

Although running and walking are both useful to promote ideal body weight, running is obviously a more concentrated exercise and takes less time. Fears that running over a period of years would lead to increased osteoarthritis and joint replacements seem to be refuted by a recent Stanford University study.[12] For many people, however, walking briskly is more enjoyable than running and less likely to aggravate prior injuries. Another option is to run with walk breaks as popularized by long distance runner, Jeff Galloway. He claims that walk breaks, e.g., one minute every mile, preserve muscle strength, decrease injuries, and enhance enjoyment of the run.[13]

REPRODUCIBILITY

The second part of Principle 7, *keep it comfortable*, is also essential to long-term activity maintenance. While weight lifting to muscle exhaustion or failure—i.e., until you simply cannot lift the weight another time—may increase muscle bulk and strength, it is too uncomfortable for me to do regularly, and I will never be on the cover of *Muscle & Fitness* magazine anyway. Likewise, doing seven-minute miles would make me anticipate my run about as much as I look forward to going to the dentist. It would be a tremendous disincentive to exercising.[14] While there is some degree of truth in the "no pain, no gain" mantra, the pain must be minimal enough so it can be sustained over years. Remember that "Too much pain, and you won't maintain."

There is no question that on some days, your exercise routine will be less than completely enjoyable, whereas on others, the time will seem to effortlessly fly by. On those off days, self-motivational thoughts can help. Remind yourself of how lucky you are to be able to be exercising. Think about how self satisfied you'll feel when you're done. Even silent "magical" chants can help, such as Jeff Galloway's suggestion to repeat over and over, "I feel good; I feel strong."[15] Sometimes it really does help.

TRAVEL

Travel poses a significant impediment to workout routines. In an effort to keep the daily exercise schedule, I recommend walking *everywhere*. Doing this may actually lead to a little weight loss on vacation, simply attributable to the extra walking that sightseeing can involve. Lightweight rain jackets, compact umbrellas, and waterproof shoes can keep you walking even in inclement weather. Many hotels have small gyms with weight lifting capabilities. Daily gym use, even in New York City, can cost as little as $20. A few sessions in a week can prevent deconditioning and make it less likely that you'll abandon your routine once you return home. Finally, packable rubber band resistance training equipment can allow you to weight lift in the privacy of your room or even your campsite. For those who think elastic bands are for weaklings, NFL All-Star Terrell Owens uses them regularly during his workouts.[16] And if you drive, you can bring along a twenty to thirty-five pound dumbbell as well.

Estimating
Calorie Burn

Wouldn't it be helpful if there were an easy way to measure exactly how many calories we expend with our daily activities and exercise regimens? A rough estimate is likely the best you'll be able to do, though, since precise measurements are only possible in research labs. Keeping records of calorie expenditure is essential if you are trying to lose weight but maintenance may require less obsessiveness. The bottom line, however, is that you must tailor your workout regimen to your specific needs. If you are trying to lose weight, your activity requirement may be higher and food intake lower than if you are simply attempting to maintain a given weight. And the intake and output balance in one person will not necessarily apply to another. You will need to experiment and adjust your intake and output for your desired individual effect.

How Intense?

Exercise physiologists and trainers like to categorize physical activity intensity by target heart rate. Your maximum heart rate can be approximated by simply subtracting your age from 220. For moderate intensity exercise, the target heart rate is 50–70% of maximum, and for vigorous intensity it is 70–85%. A forty-year-old, for example, would have a maximum of 180; a brisk walk (moderate) should get the pulse rate to between 90 and 126, and running (vigorous) between 127 and 153.

So should you buy a monitor or stop during your workout to take your pulse rate? I have never done it, but if it helps maintain your motivation, keep it up. Otherwise, try to exercise intensely enough to at least break a sweat, and remember that your ultimate target is not heart rate but, rather, your ideal body weight.

THE DOWNSIDE OF EXERCISE

Recent arguments that exercise will not help you lose weight are rather far-fetched but worth discussing. Instead of dispelling the intake and output principle, these claims reinforce it. If you work out and then go to a café for a bear claw and a cappuccino, you can obviously negate the weight reduction benefits of your exercise session. Likewise, if you sit around in a stupor all day after a workout rather than engage in your usual activities, intake and output will be adversely affected.[17] Just as in life itself, a little common sense can go a long way in your exercise regimen.

SUMMARY

In summary, regular exercise should be as much a part of your everyday routine as breathing, eating, or sleeping. It promotes weight maintenance, helps combat the inevitable stress of our modern world, results in better sleeping habits, improves self-esteem, and gives a sense of accomplishment. Regular exercise is one of the most essential keys to appearing and feeling younger than your years.

Chapter 7

BRING YOUR LUNCH

New York City now requires posting of the caloric content of menu items at chain restaurants with fifteen or more outlets. While some might feel this is like raining on the parade, examination of the numbers can be sobering. For perspective let us assume that the daily caloric intake to maintain ideal body weight is 1800 calories for a woman and for a man, 2300. The FDA recommends that daily fat intake not exceed 65 grams. A Big Mac is 576 calories with 32 grams of fat, a Whopper With Cheese,® 760 calories with 47 grams of fat, and small fries, 250 calories with 13 grams of fat. A medium soft drink is 210 calories.

So a lunch of a burger, fries, and a drink could add up to 1220 calories. This would constitute more than 60% of your recommended calories and essentially all of your recommended fat for the day! There is not much caloric room left for breakfast and dinner. Yet notice the noontime crowds at the fast food places eating this much or even more. Only an active teenager could hope to regularly eat lunch like this and not gain weight. The superficial appeal of fast food is obviously convenience and good taste at a relatively inexpensive price, but the real cost, that of weight gain and all that it entails, is steep indeed.

However, for even less money and with only slight inconvenience, you can bring your own healthy, satisfying lunch to work with markedly fewer calories than the fast food fare. I started bringing my own lunch because, ironically, the hospital dining room really didn't offer much healthy food. And furthermore, I was often busy caring for a critically ill patient during the dining room lunch hours, and then I'd snack on whatever I could find afterward.

PRINCIPLE 8

Bring a cooler.

For more than twenty-five years I have packed a lunch in a small cooler with blue ice: yogurt, granola, an apple, a pear, and a small box of raisins. While lacking variety, it is dependable, healthy, filling, and it keeps me from yielding to my hunger pangs and eating whatever is available rather than what is nutritious.

My lunch is also efficient, taking about two minutes to pack, and it can be eaten in about five minutes if time is an issue, as it often is for me. Contrast that with time spent in a midday line at McDonald's. Additionally, bringing my lunch reinforces the notion that I eat to survive and not the other way around. I will warn you, however, that your actions may brand you as a being a bit unusual if you start bringing a healthy lunch to work. Let's face it: if everyone else is eating pizza while you're having nonfat yogurt or cottage cheese for lunch, eyebrows will be raised. This may actually be beneficial, because you are essentially making a public commitment to good health and, thus, may be less inclined to cheat on your diet. Ironically, my dietary habits, at a hospital no less, are thought to be somewhat odd, as if trying to protect the only body I'll ever have is an eccentric endeavor. With a smile, I respond to this skepticism with a favorite aphorism: a sane person in an insane society appears to be insane. What is odd to me is that, as a society, we are literally eating ourselves to death.

So, let us compare the caloric burden of my usual lunch with that of the Burger King or McDonald's patron.

- Trader Joe's Greek Style Blueberry Nonfat Yogurt®—130 calories
- Granola, ¼ cup to mix in yogurt—85 calories
- One medium apple—100 calories
- One medium pear—100 calories
- One box raisins for mid-afternoon snack—130 calories

The grand total is 535 calories with 3.3 grams of fat and 15 grams of protein. For less than half of the calories and a fraction of the fat, I've had a nutritious, satisfying lunch. And to put the caloric difference into expenditure terms, my fast food counterpart would have to run more than five miles to reach caloric parity from just this one meal. Imagine the accumulation of difference in calories day after day, year after year, between the two lunches. In fact, as we shall see, a net reduction of 500 calories per day can result in a steady weight loss of one pound per week, and *this could be easily accomplished by simply switching to my lunch recipe!*

Enough about lunch. What about the other meals? Breakfast, like lunch, should be somewhat austere and low in fat. Whole grain cereal with fruit and nonfat milk or soy milk, perhaps with a small amount of chopped walnuts, can last until lunch time and provides protein, fiber, and several fruit servings. The breakdown on my typical "brekkie" (all served in one big bowl) is as follows:

- Grape Nuts,® ½ cup—200 calories
- All Bran,® ¼ cup—40 calories
- Bite sized shredded wheat, 1 cup—170 calories
- Banana, ½—70 calories
- Dried blueberries, 1/8 cup—80 calories
- Prunes, 5—100 calories
- Nonfat milk, 8 ounces—80 calories

The total is 740 calories, 2.5 grams of fat, and 22 grams of protein. My combined breakfast and lunch represent about 1300 calories, only slightly more than the fast food lunch alone and with much less fat.

For perspective, let's crunch the numbers of a Denny's Grand Slam breakfast including a small orange juice, two pancakes, two bacon strips, two sausage links, scrambled eggs, and hash browns—a Hulk-sized breakfast for sure, but not out of the ordinary at this restaurant. This represents more than 1400 calories with 76 grams of fat. How could anyone possibly eat this meal any more than once every blue moon and maintain ideal body weight?

Both breakfast and lunch should be fairly uniform from day to day.[1] Using a calorie counter booklet and reading food labels should allow you to know precisely how many calories are in your typical breakfast and lunch. For the past twenty-five years my breakfasts and lunches have varied little from what you see above, save for different flavors of yogurt and types of fruit.

PRINCIPLE 9

Be a creature of habit with a low fat,
low calorie breakfast and lunch.

Before you roll your eyes or give up on ever hoping to maintain your IBW, allow me to explain the benefits of this method. Follow the 25-25-50 rule: 25% of your total daily caloric intake for each breakfast and lunch, with 50% reserved for dinner. Lightening up the calories in the first two meals helps to prevent caloric overindulgence while allowing for a larger, more satisfying dinner. Measuring the calories of the proto-type breakfast and lunch and sticking with them on most days guarantees caloric uniformity. Get over the notion that you must have meat or other fat-laden foods three times a day. Find something healthy that you like and adhere to it. If you crave variety, measure out several breakfasts and lunches that are equivalent and that follow the 25-25-50 rule.

We humans tend to be dietary procrastinators. We may vow to eat, drink, and be merry, for tomorrow we diet, but when tomorrow comes, too many of us lose our resolve. The satiety from a large breakfast will be long gone by dinnertime. Eating light breakfasts and lunches guarantees at least partial caloric restriction.

Dinner is probably everyone's biggest meal, less rushed and more likely to be enjoyed. And if you have already exercised, worked all day, and eaten a common sense low fat breakfast and lunch, it seems reasonable to allow a little more latitude for dinner with regard to calories and fat (within limits, of course).

I recommend always having a sizable salad, which provides several servings of vegetables and is low in fat, as long as a light dressing is chosen.

PRINCIPLE 10

Use low fat salad dressing.

The difference in calories from low fat versus regular dressing can be astonishing (fifty versus 130). Regular dressing can convert what you believe is a healthy part of dinner to a calorie fest. A low fat salad before the entree helps fill the stomach with low caloric volume and helps curb your appetite for portions of your meal that may not be as healthy. In more general terms, Principle 10 emphasizes that every little bit of calorie cutting helps. Furthermore, high caloric burdens can come in unsuspected places. Read the labels.

The main dinner course should generally consist of vegetables, rice or pasta, and a small amount of lean meat or cheese for flavoring, but dinner techniques are described in more detail in Chapter 11, *Learn to Cook*. Nonfat milk as your beverage is a significant protein source without many calories. Portions should be large enough to satisfy but not huge, and the general rule should be to never have seconds, although violating this principle is occasionally permissible during a particularly active day.

Portion sizes in the United States have been gradually increasing, as have our waistlines, not only in restaurants, but at home as well. Some literal rules of thumb can be used to properly portion your dinner.

- The thumb from the first joint to the tip is about the size of an ounce of cheese or meat.
- A clenched fist is approximately one cup, or one serving of rice or pasta.
- A thumbnail is about one teaspoon.
- The size of the palm is about the equivalent of one serving or three ounces of meat.
- An ounce of nuts will fit in a cupped hand.

A calorie counting book should be in every household and assist in determining proper portions.[2,3] People who are trying to lose weight or who are having difficulty maintaining IBW will have to be more meticulous with measuring and even weighing (with a kitchen scale) their portion sizes.

A typical dinner in the Hardeman household is outlined herein, but details are provided in the Appendix.

- Vegetables and tofu, sautéed in olive oil over rice, topped with Parmesan cheese— 466 calories
- Broccoli, 1 cup —30 calories
- Salad with ¼ cup nonfat cottage cheese, ¼ cup garbanzo beans, and light dressing —290 calories
- Nonfat milk, 8 ounces—90 calories
- Dessert (Cheerios,® ½ cup topped with ½ cup fresh strawberries, 1 teaspoon sugar, and ½ cup nonfat milk)—193 calories

Dinner is about 1070 calories, bringing the daily intake tally to about 2400 calories with 80 grams of protein and 40 grams of fat. My total calorie intake may be a little higher than average because of my activity level, and you, too, will have to adjust food intake based on your own exercise patterns. Many of my patients have pointed out that an active lifestyle gives you much more leeway when it comes to the pleasure of eating.

Before writing this book, I honestly had little notion of my exact daily caloric intake. I only knew that what I was doing was maintaining my desired weight. If you are trying to lose weight, meticulously counting calories (both I&O) makes sense, but if your maintenance regimen is working, there is no urgent need to be so dedicated to the numbers. Still, you should read nutrition labels and be aware of calorically dense food. Often you should avoid certain food items because of their high calorie statistics even though you may not be keeping an Excel sheet of your I&O.

A word about tofu: it has a bad reputation in many people's eyes. I certainly acknowledge that eating a slab of soft, slimy tofu freshly retrieved from its watery package is not exactly my idea of culinary nirvana either. However, tofu now comes in firm textures that are flavored or marinated and actually taste good. It tastes best when small pieces are sautéed with vegetables in olive oil and served over rice or pasta, but adding it to sauces (e.g., marinara) also boosts protein intake, and you'll hardly even know it's there. Several years ago, when having dinner with my wife and me, my mother-in-law extracted a small piece of tofu from the casserole we were eating and asked, "Now, what kind of fish is this?" It was then that I knew that tofu could go mainstream if only people gave it a chance.

Desserts are acceptable if you are at your ideal body weight and maintaining it. But beware: all of the hard work and dietary discipline you may have exhibited during the day can be undone by one piece of chocolate cake. If you do decide to indulge in dessert, try low fat ice cream or cereal topped with fresh fruit or, better yet, fruit alone. Always wait at least twenty minutes after dinner to eat anything more, however.

PRINCIPLE 11

Wait twenty minutes after eating or snacking to eat any more.

Remember, we are genetically programmed to gorge ourselves when food is available. So sometimes our brains do not realize that we are full or overly full until we wait a little while. Snacks can be beneficial in allowing us to keep from getting excessively hungry, which can destroy our caloric willpower, but snacks must be of limited size. Cereal with nonfat milk makes an excellent snack. Sometimes a small amount of fat-containing food such as peanut butter can provide more prolonged relief of hunger pangs since fat is more slowly emptied from the stomach, but try to avoid saturated and trans fats, which increase the risk of vascular disease.

PRINCIPLE 12

Don't tempt yourself.

It is important to refrain from tempting yourself by having readily available junk food snacks around the house. If chips, cookies, and candy are present in your cupboard, they will likely eventually be eaten, so just don't buy these items. Shopping when you are hungry is likely to tempt you to purchase food you really should not have in your house. Eating just one tortilla chip or cookie is usually not possible, and sometimes it is easier to simply resist even starting. Try to alter habits associated with excessive food intake. For example, if you usually have buttered popcorn, candy, and a soda when you go to the movies, bring along your own low calorie snack instead. (Just watch out for those pesky ushers roaming the aisles!)

Part of the transformation to a healthy lifestyle involves adopting a mindset that avoids deification of food. Don't eat as entertainment.

If eating good tasting food becomes one of your hobbies, you will likely overindulge. If you return from vacation not so excited about the new sites and experiences, but rather reminiscing about how wonderful the food was, you need to re-prioritize. We eat to live, not vice versa.

It is important, however, to reward yourself from time to time by eating things simply for the pleasure of their taste. Just don't make a habit of this practice. Infrequent and responsible indulgences certainly enhance our lives, and complete Spartan denial is not likely to be conducive to long-term healthy nutritional practices. For the most part, though, avoiding food worship and adopting the mindset that nourishment is fuel will best serve you in the quest for lifelong good health.

Chapter 8

EAT PLANTS

We should all be at least part-time vegetarians. Having been a lacto-ovo vegetarian (a person who eats mostly plant-based foods in addition to eggs and dairy products but does not eat meat) for more than thirty years, I have heard the gamut of arguments against it: it's too difficult to be practical (false); it's hard to get enough protein without meat (false); you can't find anything decent on a restaurant menu (once true, now mostly false); humans evolved to be omnivores (true; arguing that canine teeth didn't develop to rip off flesh is difficult). Had our ancestors not eaten meat, none of us might be here. But in the present day there are plenty of alternative protein sources, and a plant-based diet is healthier and more likely to produce weight maintenance. Essentially, the only reason people still eat meat is for the taste—it is not necessary from a nutritional perspective in our modern world. I like to think of vegetarianism as a higher evolutionary level, often to the objection of my carnivorous friends and family members.

But, seriously, there are so many advantages to a meat free diet.

a. It is healthier. Studies have shown beneficial effects on blood pressure, cholesterol, the risk of developing cardiovascular disease and certain cancers, and survival.[1,2]

b. It is better for the animals. We are a nation of animal lovers. We pamper our dogs and cats but, curiously, eat the dead flesh of cows, pigs, and chickens.

c. It is better for the environment and a more efficient way of obtaining food. It takes up to 16 kilograms of grain and 100,000 liters of water to produce one kilogram of beef but only 2000 liters for one kilogram of soybeans. The same area of land can feed twenty times as many vegetarians as carnivores.[3,4,5]

Now, I am not advocating that everyone who reads this book become a vegetarian. It would be unrealistic to believe that readers would simply dispense with what most people consider to be an essential component of their diet. Furthermore, one can be very fit and still eat red meat, poultry, and fish. However, a predominantly plant-based diet and even a vegetarian meal or two a week may not only be healthier, but it would also keep us thinking about and trying to adhere to healthier diets. And motivation is a key factor in maintaining the AYTSA lifestyle.

Chapter 9

MY TAKE ON *MYPLATE*

ere we go again. Despite several revisions of the food pyramid in the last decade alone, the obesity epidemic's relentless march has continued. So, in June 2011, the U.S. Department of Agriculture, with the help of First Lady Michelle Obama, released its latest nutrition guidelines called MyPlate, available online at choosemyplate.gov. For many decades the U.S. government has provided information to citizens regarding healthy eating based on current scientific nutritional knowledge. The Basic Seven food groups initiated in 1943 were supplanted by a simpler Basic Four in 1956, which included meat, dairy, grains, and fruits/vegetables.[1] Notwithstanding influences from the meat and dairy industries, the recommendations were changed again in 1992 to the Food Guide Pyramid which, from its inception, has been criticized as too complicated.

Though greeted with only modest fanfare, MyPlate is meant to be the new rock star on the nutritional block, and while it may have some shortcomings, it is undoubtedly an improvement over its predecessor. Its brightly colored logo shows half of the plate taken up by fruits and vegetables with a quarter each of grains and protein. Beside it is a smaller circle labeled dairy, presumably representing a glass of milk. Protein, formerly known as the meat group, now emphasizes that meat is far from the only protein source that a healthy diet should include. There are also some simple but important recommendations below the icon, including avoiding oversized portions, switching to nonfat or 1% milk, and drinking water instead of sugary drinks.

The plate is obviously schematized since people often eat salad or fruit on a different plate, and sometimes grains, proteins, and vegetables are consumed together, such as with a hamburger. Furthermore, the icon is two dimensional, and anyone who has gone to a buffet restaurant has seen how high it is possible to stack food on a plate.

Notice that there is no place on the plate for sugars and fat-containing foods. These are relegated to the "empty calorie" category in the "Food Groups" section beneath the icon. This section, in question-and-answer format, recommends keeping empty calories to a minimum. It also does a pretty good job of describing portion amounts and practical ways of measuring them. A recurrent theme is the avoidance of excessive portion size.

Speaking of portioning your calories, this endeavor is not always that simple, but one easy way is to read the Nutrition Facts on packaged food, as is addressed on the MyPlate website. To quickly read the label, you should concentrate on serving size, servings per container, and calories per serving. Total fat and protein per serving may also be of interest, as are saturated fat and trans fat contents, and remember that the latter two are the bad fats that should be kept to a minimum. Sometimes the labels are sneaky. A candy bar, for instance, may say 120 calories per serving, but on closer inspection, you'll notice that there are two servings per container and thus 240 calories for the full bar. To add to the confusion, Nutrition Facts labels often list measurements in grams or ounces, leaving calorie counters bewildered. If the serving size of spaghetti is 2 ounces dry for 200 calories, then investing in a kitchen scale may be required. Or you could simply take out approximately one-eighth of an eight-serving package. After it is cooked, you can put it into a measuring cup, and record it for future reference. Disappointingly, a recent study using an eye-tracking camera in a simulated grocery store showed that less than 10% of shoppers looked at most of the nutrition labels on their purchases.[2] To use a dietetic metaphor, Nutrition Facts labels spoon feed us important information that we all ought to utilize to maximum advantage.

If you are maintaining your IBW while eating a healthy diet, you needn't be meticulous with calorie counting—the proof that you are doing the right thing is the stability of your weight. On the other hand, if you need to lose weight or are having difficulty maintaining IBW, counting calories will likely demonstrate that you are eating too much and reveal areas where it is easiest to cut back.

In general, MyPlate offers sound advice that can be distilled into a few sentences: Keep portion sizes honest so you don't eat too much. Drink water rather than high calorie sodas or fruit drinks. Fill yourself up with low calorie foods that are good for you, such as fruits and vegetables, and there will be less temptation to eat those that are not. Exercise regularly. Eat dessert type foods that are high in sugar and fat very sparingly.

The website is well designed and user friendly, even for those lacking computer expertise. This chapter was originally written in the pre-MyPlate era and was about simplifying the food pyramid. I listed a number of reservations about the Food Guide Pyramid at the time and was pleased to find that most of my concerns have been addressed in MyPlate. It is fun to play with, and you can even personalize your diet regimen.

Criticisms of MyPlate have already begun to surface, however, and some are perplexing. One reviewer felt that nonfat dairy should not be emphasized because milkfat is not as bad as it has been portrayed,[3] an opinion, though referenced, not shared by most registered dietitians and other nutrition experts.[4] An editorial in the *New England Journal of Medicine* complained that the recommendation to avoid sugary drinks is buried in the guidelines[5] when it is actually present on the home page.

My assessment of the drawbacks of MyPlate is a little different. Choosing foods, portions, and percentages is somewhat laborious and may be off-putting to some. Most people do not eat vegetables at breakfast. My breakfast plate is a cereal bowl, and lunch, a yogurt container, neither of which looks anything like MyPlate. The icon itself shows a very full plate and might mislead some people into oversizing their portions. Prototype meals for breakfast, lunch, and dinner with calorically equivalent substitutions would have been helpful. Easy to prepare healthy foods are not emphasized; for example, there are many healthful cold cereals, but only bran flakes are mentioned. I would have preferred that the "sugary beverages" category specified soda, fruit juices, and energy drinks since they are among the biggest contributors to our obesity problem. I would recommend that more than half of grains be whole wheat since they contain more fiber, which can lower LDL cholesterol, the so-called "bad cholesterol,"[6] and that fruit juices not be equivalent to eating fruit itself. And references to scientific articles backing up the guidelines would have been nice, since there is so much unsubstantiated material on the Internet.

My biggest criticism of MyPlate is that it does not sufficiently emphasize the importance of IBW maintenance. While I am obviously a big proponent of eating healthy foods and try to do so with my own diet, the end is much more important than the means. Someone who is obese and yet eats healthy foods is still more likely to have high blood pressure, high cholesterol, diabetes, and joint disease than another person who eats less healthy foods but maintains IBW.

Despite a few drawbacks, chooseMyPlate.gov is informative, accurate, free, and motivational and can easily be included on your computer favorites list. It offers an excellent resource for people who want to transform themselves into healthy eaters.

DON'T DRINK BEER

L ike love, alcohol can be a blessing or a curse. It can enhance
life or become a dominant master. The obvious key point is
to not over imbibe. Despite the purported health benefits of
moderate alcohol intake, I would never suggest that a non-drinker
start to drink alcohol, since a heavy drinker always starts somewhere.
Women metabolize alcohol differently than men, so they cannot safely
drink as much. The equivalent amounts of alcohol in a "drink" are
12 ounces of beer, 5 ounces of wine, and 1.5 ounces of 80 proof
distilled spirits. Men can safely consume one to two drinks, and women
one drink per day, which, in fact, may confer a health benefit. More
than that on a regular basis, however, is tempting the wrath of the gods.
Blood pressure and triglyceride levels progressively increase with three
or more drinks per day, not to mention the potential adverse effects on
the liver, brain, heart, pancreas, bone marrow, and psyche.[1,2]

A half a bottle of wine is simply too much as a daily routine.
Capping a bottle of wine after one to two glasses is the sensible
response. Furthermore, large glasses hold much more than a drink's
worth of wine or alcohol, so be honest. It's the number of ounces that
counts. The caloric content of alcoholic beverages differs considerably. Beer is the highest in calories at 150 calories per twelve ounces,
though the range extends from 70-calorie light beers to 200 calories.
Five ounces of wine is better at 130 calories. Hard alcohol is best at

100 calories, so a mixed drink with sugar-free soda or water would be the lowest calorie choice. Do not forget about alcohol as a calorie source when you crunch the numbers. Remember that fat contains 9 calories per gram while protein and carbohydrates are each 4. Alcohol is surprisingly calorie dense, weighing in at 7 calories per gram.

Imagine someone who drinks three or four beers each night on the weekends, three nights a week, which is probably not an unusual scenario. Assuming that this is an additional caloric jolt to a balanced intake and output of calories, he could potentially take in as many as 2400 additional calories per week. Since one pound of fat represents approximately 3500 calories, he could pack on as much as an extra thirty pounds in a year. Or … he could run twelve miles on Saturday and on Sunday to make up for his caloric indiscretion, an unlikely scenario. It is useful to look at foods and beverages in terms of calories you would need to expend to counteract them, and alcohol is an often-unappreciated caloric burden. Obviously, the term "beer belly" has validity, but over-consuming any alcoholic beverage can certainly lead to weight gain.

Not only is alcohol itself rich in calories, but it also decreases our inhibitions to eating calorically dense food that we might consume in more prudent portions in a non-inebriated state.

Again, judicious alcohol use can enhance life, as is the case with meat, pastries, and other traditionally unhealthy foods. Rewarding yourself occasionally may help keep you on a healthy track for the long term. But it is important to realize the tremendous levels of additional calories for which alcohol, particularly beer, may be responsible, and recall that it is all intake and output.

Chapter 11

DON'T SMOKE

This will be one of the shortest chapters in the book. Smoking cessation is non-negotiable. Everything in moderation does not apply, and unless you're one of the *Jackass* film crew, smoking is categorically, undeniably the worst thing you can do to the health of your body.

Smoking causes emphysema, chronic bronchitis, peripheral vascular disease, heart attacks, strokes, and various forms of cancer including one of the worst of all, lung cancer. And these maladies do not always lead to quick deaths; often prolonged, agonizing suffering occurs before the end.

One of the saddest moments of my medical practice was seeing a thirty-eight-year-old smoker in the office with her three young children in tow. She presented with left arm weakness and a lung mass. She ended up having lung cancer with brain metastases, a lethal diagnosis. Smokers foolishly seem to think that complications of their vice are not going to happen to them.

Not only does smoking prematurely age your internal organs, it also causes premature wrinkles. I can just about look at anyone over age forty and discern whether they smoke simply on the basis of their prominent facial wrinkles. In the medical literature, this finding has been aptly referred to as "smoker's face."[1]

If you smoke, resolve to quit today. Willpower is obviously required, but having seen hundreds of people quit, I can assure you that anyone can do it if he puts his mind to it. Those able to stop can actually experience an improvement in lung function, and this positively reinforces cessation. Nicotine replacement and various prescribed medications can help, and you may want to see your doctor. The end justifies the means, and even acupuncture and hypnosis may be of assistance, but any method necessitates a strong desire and commitment to quit. Because many people who have finally stopped smoking attempted it multiple times before, you should never quit quitting. If you think you can quit, you can, but if you think you can't, you won't. No one will ever refer to you as appearing younger than stated age if you smoke.

Chapter 12

LEARN TO COOK

Most of us can fondly recall a meal at a special restaurant where everything was perfect and delicious from the first sip of the cocktail to the last remnants of the crème brûlée. Why does restaurant food often taste so good? Well, besides the fact that we don't have to do the dishes, it is loaded with fat, calories, and salt. Everything is geared to taste, from the calorically dense salad dressing to bread and butter to entrée to decadent desserts. There is no pretense of health considerations, only taste. And that leads us to our next principle.

PRINCIPLE 13

Make eating out a special occasion.

For most of us, going out to a restaurant on a regular basis eliminates the ability to eat healthy food. There are a few tricks to help out, but healthy eating at a restaurant is just about impossible, so eating out on a regular basis should be discouraged. By one estimation, a staggering 35% of all food eaten in the United States is purchased at restaurants.[1] Dining out every two to four weeks might be reasonable, but more frequently than this is asking for caloric trouble.

The bad news is that this leaves many nights that you'll have to cook. The good news is that it is fairly easy to cook healthy, efficient, good-tasting meals that will help keep you looking and feeling young. While specific recipes can be found in the Appendix, the following are general principles that will help keep you fueled for the long run.

HEALTHY

Obviously, a major focus of preparing your own meals should be the health aspect. Generally, meals should be low in fat, especially saturated fat, and rich in vegetables, fruits, and high fiber carbohydrates. Portions should be appropriate (fist-sized) but may depend on total caloric intake and output for the day. A Spartan breakfast and lunch can allow a little more of a splurge for dinner, as might an increase in the day's physical activity. Portions also depend on weight maintenance; some people will be able to eat more than others and still maintain IBW. You will have to experiment.

SIMPLE AND QUICK

Just as with the workout, simplicity and convenience are paramount to long-lasting dietary changes. As you probably know, making everything from scratch takes too long, and a two-hour prep time won't likely bode well for permanent changes in your eating habits. A common excuse for not engaging in a healthy lifestyle is that people don't have the time. Relying on certain pre-prepared or frozen foods to which you add your personal touches is a common sense recommendation to ensure dietary compliance. Another simplicity strategy is utilizing leftovers, sometimes from two or three previous meals, for a tapas-like dinner (a la the savory snacks or appetizers served in Spanish restaurants and bars). We all have individual food preferences, and you should determine a handful of healthy fall-back dinner menus that you like to eat.

WAIT TWENTY MINUTES

Wait at least twenty minutes after dinner to have dessert to combat the biologic tendency to stuff yourself. Then have something low in fat and easy to prepare for dessert. Examples include a piece of fruit, a small amount of low fat ice cream with fruit on top, or a small bowl of cereal with fresh fruit and sprinkled with sugar. Midnight snacks or the "fourth meal," popularized by Taco Bell, are simply not conducive to long-term weight management.

PROTOTYPICAL MEAL

Specific examples are important if you are trying to transform your dietary habits. More recipes are included in the Appendix, but this meal is the prototype:

Salad: mixed greens, green onion, tomato, baby corn, garbanzo beans, ¼ cup nonfat cottage cheese with low fat dressing.

Entrée: sautéed onion, garlic, peppers, and baked tofu spooned over pasta with marinara sauce. Beverage of nonfat milk, 8 oz. side dish of vegetables such as asparagus, corn, or broccoli.

Dessert (twenty minutes later): ½ cup Cheerios with fresh berries sprinkled with sugar with nonfat milk.

This meal is obviously not steak, a baked potato, and half a bottle of red wine. At one point in my life, I liked meat and potatoes, but I don't miss them at all with healthy, satisfying meals, like the one described above.

THE RESTAURANT MEAL

Again, restaurants make their money by appealing to sense of taste, not sensibility, and the trend toward monster portions compounds the tendency to overeat. Even the energy contents of food displayed by restaurants may underestimate the true caloric load.[1] Drink sparkling water instead of alcohol. Avoid the pre-meal bread and butter. Get a salad and request dressing on the side—it is never low fat, so use it sparingly. Consider ordering an appetizer as an entrée. If portions are huge, immediately identify the easiest part of the meal to put in a doggy bag and save it to take home. Fight off the urge to order from the dessert tray and have an espresso or coffee with a little sugar instead. Oh, and in case you didn't hear me before, *don't eat at fast food restaurants.* Period.

THE OCCASIONAL REWARD

Food tastes good to us for a reason. The evolutionary advantage is self-evident. Cavemen who didn't care about eating didn't live long enough to be our ancestors. Enjoyment of food is a natural, genetic tendency, and rewarding yourself occasionally enhances life and encourages adherence to a long-term healthy diet. Contemporary circumstances, however, could easily permit us to "reward" ourselves three times a day every day, and then the reward may just become a punishment. The trick is to determine healthy foods that taste good to you and mostly stick with them.

RECIPES

The recipes included in the Appendix are meant to be a foundation to which you can add variety and adjustments to taste. They are healthy meals but not tremendously low in fat and calories, so they presume that you have eaten a sensible low fat, low calorie breakfast and lunch in accordance with the 25-25-50% program described in Chapter 7. Certainly, if you have eaten a restaurant lunch, you will need to curb the portions of dinner. *A votre santé.*

Chapter 13

UNPLUG THE TV

Watching television burns 68 calories per hour. The average U.S. household watches eight hours of TV per day. According to Web MD, Americans average twenty minutes of vigorous activity *per week*. One hour of running burns about 500 calories. I don't really need to do the math, do I? Is it any wonder that we are the United States of Obesity?

It is really impossible to live a lifestyle that embraces ideal body weight and regular exercise if discretionary time is mostly spent watching television or playing on the computer.

PRINCIPLE 14

Don't sit on your rear end.

For all their faults and excesses, television and computer entertainment may obviously enhance our awareness and knowledge. Keeping abreast of current events and being able to discuss them with others can be an important part of a mental workout (see Chapter 21). However, there is a not so subtle irony in the fact that many Americans are slowly getting fatter while watching and admiring highly trained athletes. I enjoy watching sports but rarely an entire game at one sitting and always after I have worked out myself. Passive leisure activities are fine provided you have already engaged in your daily exercises. In addition to simply observing sports, be an athlete yourself!

Not only does watching television put the caloric furnace on the low setting, it contributes to obesity in other ways as well. I couldn't even begin to estimate the average American caloric intake while in front of the TV screen—with many of us pigging out on junk food while we inertly entertain our brain cells—but it must be considerable. And we are constantly bombarded with advertisements for high calorie, good tasting food to entice us. Furthermore, staying up to watch the late late show may make us tired the next day and less likely to get up and work out.

Obviously the title of this chapter engages in hyperbole, but unlearning the habit of viewing passive entertainment is a must in order to appear younger.

Chapter 14

TAKE THE STAIRS

In the mid 1970s, at age twenty-two, I embarked upon the most exciting and transformational time of my life: starting medical school. As opposed to the celebrity worship of our current culture, it was a time when practicing physicians such as cardiac surgeons Michael DeBakey, Christian Bernard, and Denton Cooley were heroes and role models, and when the mission of becoming a doctor seemed to be the pinnacle of achievement. And there I was, leaving my home in Southern California for Baylor College of Medicine in Houston, Texas, where the school president was none other than Michael E. DeBakey himself.

I actually saw him a few times on rounds and shook his hand at my graduation ceremony. But during that time of ambition and commitment and youth that helps conjure up memories with such crystal clarity, one aspect of Dr. DeBakey is most vivid in my mind. He used to have a legion of followers when he made rounds at the Methodist Hospital: nurses, medical students, interns, residents, and fellows all trailed behind him, stopping for visits at various patients' bedsides. And, famously, DeBakey liked to take the stairs, his serpentine entourage in tow.

His wife of many years had died some time before I started at Baylor. While I was in medical school an announcement was made that DeBakey, in his mid sixties, was getting married to an actress many decades his junior. A second announcement came, months after the first: his new wife was pregnant. While some of my fellow medical students were joking and smirking, I was having an epiphany. *From now on*, I vowed, *I'm taking the stairs.*

PRINCIPLE 15

Take the stairs whenever possible.

Taking the stairs over the years has served me well, as it did Dr. DeBakey, who was still practicing medicine until his death in 2008, just months shy of his one hundredth birthday. Befittingly, his initials spelled MED. The point of taking the stairs is that every little bit of activity that you do on a daily basis adds up to help create a caloric balance and maintain an ideal body weight. Even fidgeters, of which I am one, burn more calories than those who sit still.[1] So when you're at your desk, you might just try bouncing your leg up and down a little. Every calorie counts.

Several years ago a campaign was launched to encourage folks to walk 10,000 steps per day with a pedometer, the theory being that if people know how much they have walked in a given day, they may be motivated to go farther to reach the 10,000 steps or five mile goal.[2] Every step you take, whether it's shopping in the grocery store or climbing the stairs at work, burns calories. Importantly, exercise does not need to be continuous to have beneficial effects. Three ten-minute walks spread throughout the day are calorically equivalent to one thirty-minute walk.[3] And even going downstairs expends more energy than walking on a flat surface. As an added bonus, taking the stairs for six flights or fewer often takes about the same time or less than an elevator. There has even been a mini-study in the medical literature indicating that stair-walkers saved fifteen minutes each workday compared with those who took the elevators.[4] Free time *and* free exercise in one activity!

So get a pedometer if you'd like, but look for any occasion to increase caloric expenditure in your daily life. If you work on the twentieth floor, take the elevator to the fifteenth and climb the stairs the rest of the way. Walk up and down escalators. Avoid people movers at the airport. Park a little farther away, and walk when you go to the store; don't be that person who sits for five minutes in the car waiting for a closer parking space. If you talk on the phone a lot, try to walk around during conversations. Stroll the sidelines during your daughter's soccer game instead of sitting. Ride a stationary bicycle or exercise your arms with dumbbells while watching television. The American Dietetic Association relates that while watching two hours of prime time TV, one client logged thirty minutes on her stationary bike by just pedaling during the commercial breaks.[5] Walk quickly with a spring in your step and try to never lose it. Try to walk more and drive less. Be imaginative, and you'll find all kinds of opportunities to burn a few extra calories here and there.

An eighty-eight-year-old patient of mine, a trim woman who volunteers at the hospital, told me—when I inquired about her ability to care for herself—that she walks about five miles a day during her volunteer shift. "I've always been active," she confided, "and that's the way I'll stay." In fact, when I have asked young-looking older patients to reveal their secrets, the overwhelming majority of them have said the same thing: *stay active.* Activity seems to begat activity; activity perpetuates itself. A friend who taught me to snowboard seventeen years ago owned a carpet company before retiring. He has always been active and told me that when someone came to talk to him about a work related problem, he often suggested that they go for a walk while they discussed the situation. He's now a month shy of his eightieth birthday and still rips down the mountain on his snowboard, an active role model for us all.

Every bit of activity that you do during the day, regardless of how trivial, helps to burn more cumulative calories than being inert, so use your imagination with everyday activities, and cultivate for yourself an active lifestyle.

Chapter 15

HAVE A YEARLY GOAL

For the past ten years, my wife and I have scheduled a long hike in Yosemite National Park during the late summer. Most often Half Dome, a sixteen-mile, one-day round trip trek, has been our destination, and we have not been alone in our tradition; we met a man in his seventies a few seasons ago who was making his twentieth annual Half Dome ascent.

PRINCIPLE 16

Have a physical endurance goal each year.

The hike is beautiful but challenging, exciting but exhausting, and we eagerly look forward to it with both anticipation and a little trepidation each year. One day of vigorous activity is, of course, not transformational. But the distance necessitates forced training; if we did not prepare for such a long hike for several months beforehand, we likely could not finish it. With such a goal, whether it be a long hike, bicycle ride, running or walking a half marathon, or an abbreviated triathlon, having a goal motivates one to adopt a more active lifestyle. Each summer my wife and I train to prepare for the Yosemite hike, and those fitness habits spill over into the rest of the year.

The ability to train the human body is one of its many miracles. Untrained, you might struggle to run a mile or two with a racing heart and sore muscles, but within six to eight weeks of training, you can breeze through a few miles much more effortlessly. The body obviously changes in response to regular exercise. Aerobic activities, those that involve oxygen consumption by the body, include submaximal walking, running, bicycling, and swimming. Anaerobic exercise, which includes weight training and rapid short-distance running, requires sudden bursts of strenuous activity. It is not as dependent on oxygen but cannot usually be sustained for long periods like aerobic exercise can. The two processes work via different metabolic pathways but may be thought of as two points on the exercise spectrum. For example, a runner could transition from jogging (aerobic) to sprinting (anaerobic) back to jogging (aerobic again) in the same workout session.

Aerobic exercise promotes improvement in the efficiency of heart function. During exercise, the heart must intensify the delivery of blood and oxygen to the muscles. Training improves this function by increasing stroke volume, the amount of blood pumped per heartbeat. To accomplish this, the heart contracts with greater force and empties its chambers more completely. This provides more blood flow to the exercising muscles and decreases the need for the heart to race as fast.[1]

As far as the muscles are concerned, physical endurance training is exercise-type specific.[2] In other words, if you are training for a long bike ride, you must train by bicycling—running or walking will not adequately train the biking muscles. Just as the heart becomes more efficient from training, so do the specific muscles. The tiny blood vessels, called capillaries, actually increase in number so more blood can flow to the muscles. Exercised muscles become larger so they can better endure the specific exercise. And the subcellular energy factories of the muscle cells, called mitochondria, actually increase in size and efficiency so that more energy can be generated per muscle cell.[3]

Besides a yearly goal, it helps to develop activity-related hobbies. I like to think of exercising as one of my hobbies, but I also participate in enjoyable activities that help burn calories. Hiking, biking, gardening, tennis, racquetball, golf (walking the course), skiing, and swimming are simply better activities to embrace than crocheting, wood carving, or bird watching when it comes to caloric balance.

Much of adopting and maintaining a healthy lifestyle is motivation. If you are defined by your lifestyle, this self-identity helps keep you motivated. So let people know about your yearly goal. Making a public stand can help incentivize your objectives, though others will love to criticize any unhealthy forays that you may make. When people point at me with feigned shock when I occasionally eat a piece of chocolate, I explain that I may be a health nut, but I'm a practical health nut. I believe that periodic rewards actually help me maintain a healthy lifestyle for the long run. But I thank them for pointing out my lapses into hypocrisy because this keeps me motivated as well. If you adopt the AYTSA protocol, you will influence others, which provides further motivation.

The yearly goal necessitates dedication to training, so I suggest that you do it with a spouse, your family, a friend, or a group of friends. That way there is an interpersonal responsibility for completing the task: shared training, shared motivation, and the most important aspect of returning next year for the goal, a sense of shared accomplishment.

The last several hundred yards of the Half Dome hike involves the steep ascent of a huge face of granite, pulling one's self up a 45-degree angle with cables.[4] During our first few trips my wife declined to participate in this final part of the upward trek. Finally, in 2004, she ratcheted up her courage to make the entire hike. The mutual feeling of achievement was intoxicating. It remains one of the best days of our lives and keeps us coming back each year to repeat our annual goal.

Chapter 16

BEN FRANKLIN REDUX

I cannot begin to count the number of times that patients have told me that they would like to work out, to adopt a healthier lifestyle, but they just don't have the time. Not really true, I tell them. Everyone has the time; it's simply how you prioritize it. I've already shown you that packing a nutritious lunch takes less time than waiting in line at McDonald's. Or how taking the stairs instead of the elevator often utilizes the same or even less time.

As a physician, I have often worked sixty to one hundred-hour weeks and somehow fit in an exercise regimen, so I know others can do it as well. We all budget time in our days for essentials such as work and sleep, and I'm simply saying that you need to set aside time for exercise as well. Efficient time management is essential to providing the opportunity for exercise. And from many years of experience, I believe the best way to do this is to rise early to work out. This way you will not have that obligation looming over you all day—it will already be done. And, of course, rising early will necessitate going to bed early. (Finally, the Ben Franklin reference!)

PRINCIPLE 17

Early to bed, early to rise,
helps you maintain your ideal body size.

As a further incentive to adopt this lifestyle change, most people do not participate in healthy habits after eight or nine at night. They don't usually exercise, do housework, or take part in activity related hobbies. More likely they engage in sedentary activities like watching television, eating, or reading. They might go out to a restaurant, a movie, or a bar. And with the exception of dancing, none of these activities helps to maintain a favorable caloric balance. When people substitute sleeping in for working out and staying up late for sleeping ... well, 67% of Americans become overweight.

Obviously, some people find it easier to be early risers than others. It is not clear as to what makes one a "morning" or an "evening" person, but these differences may be explained by individual circadian rhythms. Circadian literally means "about the day" and refers to the many twenty-four-hour rhythms that occur in humans. The most obvious is the sleep-wake cycle, but there are also variations in hormone levels, body temperature, internal organ function, and neuropsychiatric status depending on the time of day.[1]

Since our ancestors were dependent upon sunlight for pursuit of food, they probably started early in the morning to ensure that they had secured nutrition by the time darkness fell. One could argue that this might have given a genetic advantage to early risers; thus, perhaps we are all evolutionarily programmed to be morning people. Certainly genetic and environmental factors play a role, but evidence suggests that adhering to a routine and light exposure can alter individual circadian rhythms so that evening and morning tendencies can be potentially reversed.[2]

Experts vary in their recommendations for optimum workout times. Research has shown that peak performance may occur in the afternoon, yet other studies have refuted this notion.[3,4] According to some experts, those who work out in the morning are more likely to adhere to their regimens.[5] Interestingly, there may be a circadian specificity to your workout time, so if you are planning to run a marathon that begins at seven a.m., you might benefit by training at this time of day as well.[6]

Personal observation has led me to hypothesize another reason to engage in morning exercise. I have noticed that afternoon workouts tend to be a little more painful for me. During a good portion of my morning runs, I often feel as if I'm still half-asleep, and I believe that this dulls the pain a little bit. The grogginess and impaired cognition that we experience after awakening has been termed "sleep inertia" which, in some people, may last for several hours.[7] While far from scientifically proven, we should utilize every method possible to stay motivated, and, perhaps, using this trance-like sleep inertia period to exercise may help.

Another potential advantage to an early morning workout regimen involves what psychologist Roy Baumeister has termed "ego depletion."[8] Although willpower can be strengthened by repeated use, it can also be fatigued by overuse. The multiple decisions that we must all make during our workdays require self-discipline which can essentially be used up by the end of the day, thereby impairing adherence to an after-work exercise program. Get it done early before your steely resolve has waned.

Again, I strongly believe in a practical approach to fitness, and if you can successfully work out in the afternoon or evening and adhere to it on a long-term basis, then keep it up. Fitting the workout into each day is the most important concept, even if your schedule requires you to do it at various times of the day. For most people, however, I think that early to exercise and early to bed confers the greatest success of a lifelong exercise pattern.

Chapter 17

WEIGHT LOSS

owing your lawn when it has grown half an inch is much simpler than waiting until the grass is waist high. By the same token, deciding to embark on a weight loss program when you can pinch only half an inch around your waist—rather than waiting until you've grown unsightly love handles—is the wiser choice. I make no guarantees that reading this chapter will allow you to happily skip along the road to reduction of your body mass. Weight maintenance is more straightforward and less painful, but no such claim can be made for weight loss. There is no easy way. The fad diets, the celebrity endorsed methods, even the surgical approaches rely on one principle and one principle only: it's all I&O. Hopefully this concept is familiar to you since we discussed it extensively in Chapter 4, but it is the de facto theme of this book and bears repeating. In accordance with the I&O principle, there are three key mechanisms in weight loss/maintenance:

- Diet, i.e., restricting caloric intake enough.
- Physical activity, i.e., burning enough calories.
- Behavioral factors, i.e., convincing oneself to adhere to the appropriate dietary and physical activity strategies.

Weight gain and obesity, of course, are very complex occurrences and are influenced by individual metabolic, genetic, behavioral, and environmental factors. Therefore, some people are going to have more difficulty losing weight and maintaining their ideal body weight than others. However, as we have discussed, famine spares no one—everyone loses weight. Likewise, surgical techniques work by limiting the amount of food that the stomach can hold, or in times past, intestines were re-routed to promote malabsorption of food. In other words, these operations limit the amount of food to which the body has access, producing an obligatory weight reduction diet. The same effect can be attained by simply decreasing food intake but without the abdominal incisions.

DIETARY NIHILISM

The inherent stumbling block to losing weight is building the willpower to resist the urge to eat. I have noticed a trend in the media of late that I refer to as dietary nihilism. With so much good tasting, calorically dense food and so many activity saving devices available, some people are saying it is basically a hopeless endeavor to lose weight and keep it off. One researcher went so far as to opine that only with a massive community program to ensure good health is there a chance that we can adopt healthy lifestyles.[1]

I certainly do not subscribe to this abrogation of personal responsibility. To essentially give up when it comes to weight control is an insult to our ancestors who endured hardships that we can only imagine in order to deliver our DNA to us. Humans are blessed with reason and free will, and weight loss is certainly within our ability. Applying the victim mentality to obesity will guarantee failure in trying to reverse the situation.

Everyone has the ability to lose weight, but it will not necessarily be easy. It requires great dedication and a personal transformation along with an obsessiveness that might previously have been channeled into overeating. As stated above, weight loss will be easier for some than others. Older people who have more age and weight related joint damage will be less able to exercise and will encounter more difficulty losing weight. Thus, delaying this endeavor only lessens your chance for success. There is no better time to start your transformation than today.

WEIGHT LOSS/WEIGHT MAINTENANCE

There are two parts to weight reduction: losing the weight and maintaining the weight loss. A surge of motivation often makes the actual weight loss possible, only to see a gradual return of the pounds as motivation wanes. Theoretically, maintenance should be easier, since the ratio of intake to output of calories does not need to be as severely reduced. In reality, however, it does seem that formerly obese people who lose weight often have trouble keeping it off.[2]

Once the target weight has been attained, constant vigilance and immediate intervention to eliminate any slight weight gain are required. The hypothesis that once you become overweight there is a new "set point" in the brain that adjusts the appetite upward is unproven, and regaining lost body weight is more likely related to decreased physical activity.[3] To reiterate, regular exercise is particularly important in maintaining the weight loss that you worked so hard to achieve.[4] For most people it is likely easier to maintain IBW if they have never gained too much weight in the first place. The formerly obese must vow never to go through the weight loss phase again. Behavioral factors are obviously a huge part of both aspects of weight loss.

PRINCIPLE 18

One pound of fat = 3500 calories.

Although somewhat of an oversimplification, it is useful to think about weight loss in I&O terms. A pound of fat represents approximately 3500 calories. At a reasonable weight loss rate of one pound per week, you must expend 500 more calories per day than you take in. Of course, this assumes that your caloric balance was maintaining your weight at a steady state. If you were slowly gaining weight at about a pound a month, that would translate into about 110 extra calories taken in per day (3500 divided by thirty days). To lose a pound a week, you would then have to expend 610 more calories per day than you take in.

Improving your caloric ratio to lose weight can be accomplished by any combination of decreased food intake and increased activity. The extremes, of course, would be cutting back on daily consumption by 500 calories (eliminate one Big Mac per day) or exercising an additional 500 calories (running five miles a day). The healthiest and most practical approach is to do both, e.g., cut 250 calories from your daily meals and run 2.5 miles.

The 500-calorie rule, again, assumes no other behavioral changes that would affect weight balance. For example, a man who runs three miles but works up a thirst and drinks two cans of regular soda has just negated all the caloric effects of his exercise. Likewise, someone who markedly restricts food intake but also decreases her usual daily activity might not experience the desired weight loss.

As much as we would all like weight loss to conform to an exact science, that it will never do. Part of the problem is determining just how many calories are in each forkful of food or how much energy is burned doing forty minutes of yard work. Naturally, amounts of calories will depend upon the size and components of the forkful or the intensity of the yard work.

For this reason I encourage dieters to eat foods and do exercises that are easier to calorically quantify. Get a calorie counter, look at the food labels, measure carefully, and be honest about portion sizes. As far as activity is concerned, walking or running are the easiest to measure. This way, you can assess caloric exchanges: for example, eating a candy bar would be the equivalent of running 2.5 miles. On the other hand, if you do a nine-mile hike, the candy bar might not be so unreasonable. As always, however, practicality rules, so if your inexact intake and output of calories is leading to successful weight loss, continue it.

WHAT WE CAN LEARN FROM THE NATIONAL WEIGHT CONTROL REGISTRY

Although much obesity research has been done, the best methods for weight loss and maintenance have been elusive. Any program that works invokes the intake and output principle, but the optimum method may vary from person to person. Some generalizations have been established, however. A restricted calorie diet combined with regular exercise seems to be more effective than either alone, and exercise may be essential for weight maintenance. People who are given precise dietary components may do better than those with a self-directed diet. And those who join a weight loss program with friends are more likely to be successful than those who enroll alone.

Certain people are able to not only lose weight, but also to maintain that loss, and we can learn from their experiences. The National Weight Control Registry (NWCR) was started in 1994 to be an ongoing study of long-term successful weight reduction. To be included, subjects need to be older than eighteen and have lost thirty pounds and maintained that level for at least one year. There are more than 3000 participants in the registry; they have lost an average of sixty pounds, and they have kept it off for more than six years!

Here are some important aspects of their success:

- First of all, it is important to acknowledge that these people exist. It *is* possible to lose weight and maintain it. Thousands have done it.
- Those who succeeded had many times before attempted to lose weight but to no avail. Unsurprisingly, the success was attributable to greater dietary constraint and more exercise. In the words

of Winston Churchill, "Never, ever, ever, give up." (Author's note: Actually, there is controversy as to exactly how many "nevers" and "evers" are in this quotation. I'm pretty sure Sir Winston wasn't referring to dieting, but, nonetheless, it applies to this NWCR data, which hopefully will serve as an inspiration to millions of frustrated dieters.)

- They ate low calorie, low fat diets, averaging less than 1500 calories per day, 24% of which was from fat. Less than 1% used a low carb, Atkins-type diet.
- Half lost weight under supervision, and half did it on their own.
- They regularly ate five small meals per day. Almost 80% ate breakfast, and they consumed less than one meal per week at a fast food restaurant.
- They exercised a lot: 2800 calories of exercise per week, which, in walking terms, represents more than 4 miles a day. They averaged 1-1.5 hours of exercise per day.
- Almost all participants felt that weight loss had enhanced their lives, resulting in more energy, higher self-confidence, better ability to be active, and improved emotional state.[5]

Using NWCR information, along with the principles from this book, I have assembled some recommendations for those embarking on a weight loss program.

RULES OF ENGAGEMENT FOR WEIGHT LOSS

1. Lifestyle transformation is essential.
2. Set a date. Don't try to start your diet during the holiday season, on your birthday, or the day of the company picnic where temptation may overwhelm good intentions. Try to psych yourself up for the start date. Studies suggest that self-discipline may be like a muscle: the more you use it, the stronger it gets.

3. Empty your household of all temptation food.

4. Write down everything you eat, its estimated calories, your structured exercise, and approximate caloric expenditures. People tend to overestimate caloric expenditure and underestimate their intake, and writing it down helps to keep you honest. A reasonable weight loss goal of one pound per week requires the net loss of 500 calories per day and is most reasonably approached by restricting your diet by 250 calories and exercising an additional 250 calories.

5. Be honest about your portions. An entire plate of pasta could have four times the calories of what is considered a normal size portion: the size of your fist. Some wine glasses can contain 15 ounces, about three times a normal serving. Measure, read nutritional labels, and utilize your calorie counter booklet.

6. Have available low fat snacks. Sliced vegetables, nonfat cottage cheese, nonfat Greek yogurt (lower in calories and higher in protein than traditional nonfat yogurt), and hard-boiled egg whites are good examples. Put snack-sized portions in ziplock bags for easy portability and access.

7. Review *ZPG* and *Use the Stairs* chapters.

8. Absolutely avoid the following foods while you are trying to lose weight. Whether you can consume these sparingly when on the maintenance phase will depend upon the individual.

   a. Fast food of any sort.

   b. Soda, sports drinks, fruit juices, and energy drinks (sugar-free sodas are obviously permissible). Sugar-filled beverages could be unique in that they might slip past the calorie detection mechanism of the body.[6] Given that evolution has really only dealt with one beverage for most of humanity's existence—that is, water—sugary drinks may pack in the calories without making you feel full. Even in the maintenance phase, these liquid candies should be avoided. Instead, drink what your ancestors did: water.

    c. Alcohol—if you enjoy one drink or less per day, you can probably reinstitute such a habit in the maintenance phase.

    d. Dessert, except for fresh fruit.

    e. Donuts and all other deep fried foods.

    f. Free food. Muffins in the break room at work or samples in grocery stores may be tempting and free, but they're anything but calorie free.

    g. Second helpings —no elaboration necessary.

    h. Restaurant food. Avoid this altogether during the weight loss phase if you can. If you must go out for social reasons, see *Learn To Cook* chapter for tips in healthy restaurant eating.

9. Always wait at least twenty minutes after a meal or snack before deciding that you're hungry enough to eat more. As we've previously seen, there can be a cephalo-gastric disassociation that encourages us to gorge on food. The hunger center of the brain lags behind the stomach when it comes to satiety. Waiting twenty minutes often allows us to appreciate that we were full after all.

10. Exercise at least 1 ½ to 2 hours per day. Yes, you read it right, 90-120 minutes per day. See *Workout* and *Take the Stairs* chapters. Start gradually and work your way up. See your doctor first for approval.

11. If you are overweight and experience marked fatigue during the day, a treatable medical disorder may be present. See your doctor for a simple blood test to check thyroid function, although only a small minority of overweight people actually has hypothyroidism. If you snore at night and have daytime sleepiness, you could have sleep apnea, which is very common. This disorder can cause profound sleep deprivation and make it difficult to think straight, let alone exercise every day. Again, see your doctor if you think you might have sleep apnea.

12. Arthritis, emphysema, heart disease, or any other condition that limits mobility will complicate weight loss because exercise is more

difficult. Often the early stages of weight reduction will depend primarily on calorie restriction. However, even the loss of 10% of body weight can significantly improve physical capabilities and allow increasing activity to contribute to the weight loss cause. Certainly, if you have heart or lung disease, check with your doctor before starting an exercise program.

13. People who have recurrently tried, unsuccessfully, to lose weight with a BMI more than 40 should consider contacting their physicians regarding possible pharmacological or surgical options, the discussion of which is beyond the intent of this book.

14. Once you have reached IBW, *never leave it*. Caloric restrictions can be relaxed but never completely discarded since your goal is now to maintain current weight, not lose any more. However, you must weigh yourself daily, and if there is a 5% increase from your ideal body weight, address it immediately with the steps delineated above.

SUMMARY

Weight loss *can* be accomplished even if you've tried many times before, though it requires discarding old habits and embracing a new lifestyle. Patience is required, and the one pound per week/500 calories per day formula is realistic and sustainable. While requiring a less strict application of the intake and output principle, weight maintenance, as opposed to weight loss, is forever and requires constant vigilance. Even in the maintenance phase, this chapter will be useful to combat any upward deviation of your IBW; nip it in the bud before your body fat blossoms. And remember that, like muscle, you may be able to bulk up your self-discipline by simply using it more.[7,8]

Chapter 18

GETTING STARTED

G etting started is always the hardest part. Dispensing with our prior lifestyles and habits and adopting new, healthier principles of living will take effort. But as the fruits of our labors become evident, healthy living becomes easier and finally just becomes a part of us. This chapter is about the specific first steps to get the transition started.

1. Take off all of your clothes, stand in front of the mirror, and make a vow to transform yourself so that healthy living becomes part of your self-identity. Take a good look because you may never see that same reflection again.

2. Buy a scale, weigh yourself, calculate your IBW, and compare the numbers. Design a plan to get to your IBW by one pound per week or 500 calories net loss per day.

3. Empty your kitchen pantry of all junk and temptation foods including chips, sodas, pastries, candy, cookies—and, yes, beer.

4. Go grocery shopping. Stock up on pasta, rice, tofu, cereals, olive oil, low fat salad dressing, nonfat yogurt, granola, and fresh fruit and vegetables. A word about milk: most people who drink whole milk view the nonfat variety as thin, watery, and unappetizing, whereas nonfat drinkers look at whole milk as thick, fatty, and disgusting. It's all what you get used to, and transitioning to nonfat is easy. Drink 2% for one month, 1%

for one month; then, create a mixture to equal 0.5% for one month; finally, graduate to completely nonfat, and you'll never go back.

5. Buy a calorie counter booklet, and start closely inspecting food nutrition labels.

6. Buy a small cooler and blue ice so you can bring your lunch to work.

7. Purchase two pairs of running/walking shoes. One-hundred-dollar shoes are not necessary. Discount outlets and discontinued models provide high quality shoes for a reasonable price. Alternating your pairs of shoes may allow the cushion to re-expand between uses, thereby prolonging the life of the shoes. Map out a course for your walk in your neighborhood. A one or two mile loop that goes by your house is often convenient. That way you can leave a water bottle on your front porch and have a place to make a pit stop if nature calls.

8. Get a pedometer. This way you can assess how many steps your day-to-day activities require. The 10,000 steps goal is a worthy one. Scientific studies have indicated that using a pedometer actually encourages an increase in daily walking distances.[1]

9. Buy a weight bench and weights. See Appendix for specific techniques.

10. Find a book of local hikes in your area. Hiking is one of the most convenient activity-related hobbies. A minimum of equipment is required, it can be done almost anywhere, and it will take you places you might never have otherwise seen. And a long destination hike makes an excellent yearly goal.

Chapter 19

STAYING MOTIVATED

Y ou're at your ideal body weight. You may just be in the best shape of your life. You exercise regularly and eat sensibly. So what now? Stay motivated!

When it comes to physical fitness, there is no destination. There is only the journey. In a period of months, even the most physically fit person can become fat and lazy if he loses his motivation, and thus, good health requires eternal vigilance.

REJOICE IN YOUR FITNESS

When initiating a fitness program, patience is essential. You will likely not see significant changes in your body for several months. Once you do notice that you are trimmer and fitter, the positive feedback your efforts elicit from friends and family can keep the motivation flowing. It's okay to revel in the healthier you; the more pleasure and pride you derive from being fit, the more you will be driven to stay that way. You can even privately feel superior to others as long as it helps to maintain your motivation.

KEEP IT SIMPLE AND COMFORTABLE

Principle 7, again. Both your diet and exercise regimen must be sustainable for a lifetime. Despite my recommendations, I have a friend who is in a continuous boom and bust pattern with his workouts. Once motivated, he tries to progressively increase his running distance. What starts out as a few miles a day turns into an arduous six miles or more, at which point he usually loses his motivation and reverts back to an exercise-free existence. To use an appropriate metaphor, remember that your workout regimen is a marathon and not a sprint—design it for the long run.

Self-identity

If you work on convincing yourself that regular exercise is an essential part of you for long enough, it will become so. The transformation to a healthy lifestyle needs to be both in the muscles and in the brain. A healthy, fit person will not only be what you are, it will be who you are. Try to make yourself feel guilty if you fail to exercise or stray from your diet. And, in turn, enjoy the pride and self-esteem that regular exercising brings.

Find a Partner

My wife has an early morning walking partner, and I notice that when her partner is not able to walk, my wife is less likely to go as well. Conversely, she feels she has a responsibility to be there if someone else is depending on her. So, if it motivates you, find an exercise partner with whom there is a mutual responsibility for maintenance of your workout regimen.[1] However … the most reliable, dependable person to keep you motivated is yourself. Don't dispense with your exercise plans just because someone else doesn't show up. Always be prepared to work out by yourself.

Get a Dog

There is an exception to the paragraph above. A dog will never fail to accompany you on a walk in favor of sleeping in. Many of my patients have reported losing weight thanks to their canine companions.

KEEP DOING THE FUN THINGS

Often during a workout or run I occupy my mind by thinking about how exercise allows me to keep doing the fun things in life. It may be four months before ski season begins, but yet I imagine snowboarding through steep and deep powder, one of the best feelings in the world, and my pace picks up. Regular exercise will keep you in the condition required to play a vigorous set of tennis or ski down a black diamond or hike to the top of a mountain. Not only do fun activities motivate exercise, but the converse is also true. When you know that your muscles are well conditioned and that you won't be hobbling around after a basketball game, you'll be more likely to participate.

GET AN MP3 PLAYER

Although I have been exercising regularly for more than four decades, a now essential part of my routine is something I've had for only six years: my iPod. Studies showing that we are genetically programmed to derive meaning from music are consistent with the motivation it confers upon exercisers.[2] With my iPod on shuffle, I notice that my stride quickens when a favorite song begins. For me, this might be something by the Rolling Stones, Iron Maiden or Rise Against. But whether it's Metallica, Manilow, or Mozart, you can program a personal adrenalin soundtrack to keep yourself fully amped. Putting auditory ambition to work for you is part of exploiting every advantage in your war against poor health.

Just be cautious with the volume. Cranking it up for a song or two may be okay, but prolonged loud music delivered so directly to your ears may damage hearing irreversibly.[3] You don't want to have to say, "Eh?" when someone is complimenting you on your youthful appearance.

DISTINGUISH YOURSELF

Most of us have never been hoisted on the shoulders of our team-mates after making the victorious touchdown run. Few of us have heard the crowd go wild after we have shot the winning buzzer-beater on the basketball court. By definition, the majority of us are average. We can, however, distinguish ourselves by staying fit regardless of any God-given athletic talent. Dedication and determination are the only requirements. And instead of a fleeting victory dance, we can derive self-satisfaction from physical fitness that lasts a lifetime.

INTAKE AND OUTPUT

Here it is again: I&O. As we've discussed, one of the problems with caloric balance is that it's so much quicker and easier to take in lots of calories than it is to expend them. Even the leisurely consumption of a 360-calorie muffin takes less than ten minutes. Contrast that with the 35-40 minutes of running or 55 minutes of walking to burn those same 360 calories. Start to look at foods within the framework of how many calories you'll need to work them off. To use a financial metaphor, the muffin is lending you 360 calories that you must pay back in exercise if you hope to maintain your ideal body weight.

Exercising regularly does not grant you license to eat indiscriminately or to become more torpid than usual for the remainder of the day. Try to develop a mind-set that exercise is its own reward. You don't need to treat yourself to a doughnut after a workout, or coddle yourself by not taking the stairs later in the day. The I&O principle mandates that every little bit of extra activity helps and every extra morsel of food hurts your efforts to maintain ideal body weight. A recent *TIME* magazine cover article proposes an "exercise myth"—claiming that exercise doesn't lead to weight loss.[4] While superficially ridiculous, their contention that some people overeat or become underactive after exercising is well taken.

GO THE DISTANCE, NOT THE SPEED

Inevitably, there will be some days that you just don't feel up to going full force with your workout. Maybe you're a little under the weather, or perhaps you didn't get enough sleep the night before. Under these circumstances, try to get your exercise done but at a slower pace. Take more walk breaks if you're running or go slower if you're walking. The more time off you take from exercising, the more painful it will be to resume, and pain can be a motivation killer.

When you're ill, bed rest may be unavoidable, especially if you feel like vomiting your insides up or if you're having fever and chills from influenza. But for the most part, we physicians do not recommend bed rest for *anything* anymore—not for back pain, not for the flu, not even after surgery. Even open-heart patients usually go for their first walk within twenty-four hours of their surgery. In 1992, I contracted tuberculosis from a patient and had to take a few weeks off until medications rendered me non-communicable.[5] Though I was a bit tired, I continued to run and exercise like normal. Staying active and adhering to your routine, even if some days are a little slower, helps keep you motivated to stay the course.

BE A ROLE MODEL

Leading by example is one of the best ways to influence others. Everyone wants his or her family to be healthy. Teach and encourage your children to engage in and appreciate exercise. As we have discussed, there is some evidence that the more active they are at a young age, the healthier they will be later. Adopt the "do as I say and as I do" mantra as a responsibility not only to yourself but also to your loved ones, and soon your entire family will be healthier.

SELF-DISCIPLINE: USE IT OR LOSE IT?

Psychology is starting to seriously devote research to aspects of human behavior that were never studied before. Happiness, self-esteem, and procrastination are examples of modern psychology research topics that are becoming more fully understood. Self-discipline—or as researchers are now calling it, self-regulation—is another such subject and has been shown to perhaps be a better predictor of success than IQ. Personalities obviously differ, but self-discipline appears to be within everyone's capability and may be strengthened with repeated use, thus the analogy to building muscle. There are those who claim, however, that, like muscle, self-discipline can be fatigued by overuse, so pushing yourself too hard could possibly be counterproductive.[6,7]

I have encountered both of these aspects of self-discipline in my medical practice. Those patients who begin by cutting calories often seem to be more motivated to exercise and vice versa. On the other hand, boom and bust exercisers often pursue so much activity that self-discipline becomes overwhelmed, and good intentions are abandoned. Further studies may elucidate these issues, but for now it seems reasonable to practice common sense self-discipline until it is strong enough to become incorporated into your personality. The stronger your self-discipline, the better you will be motivated to achieve healthy dietary and exercise habits.

DEALING WITH HUNGER

Sight, smell, hormone release, habits, psychological input, and availability influence our sense of hunger, among many other factors. Just knowing that there are cookies in your pantry could lead to a consumption orgy, so calorie-proof your house by eliminating these temptations. Substitution is key; have readily available low fat, low calorie snacks at hand rather taking that first cookie. The one pound per week or 500 calorie per day weight loss program is gradual enough that no one is likely to feel that she's starving. If you do experience hunger, guard against overeating. Eat just enough to take the edge off of hunger and then stop. Volumetrics may help; keeping the stomach feeling full with high fiber, low calorie, water-containing foods may delay gastric emptying and improve satiety.[8] If you have a tendency to gorge at mealtimes, consider two recent studies that found that participants who ate an apple or drank sixteen ounces of water before meals took in fewer total calories.[9,10] And remember that while our ancestors associated hunger with the real threat of starvation, we can calmly realize that our next meal is assured.

END THE MEAL

If you never stop eating, you will never be able to maintain your ideal body weight, so you must develop strategies to *end the meal.* The brain may require about twenty minutes to receive the intestinal message that you are actually already full, so engaging in activities that finalize the meal can help prevent postprandial snacking. Brushing your teeth or chewing sugarless gum may help. Better yet, do something a little more labor intensive that you really don't want to immediately repeat: floss. After dinner alcoholic drinks are a particularly bad idea, not only because they are calorically dense; they also encourage an if-it-feels-good-do-it attitude toward eating. Try to reason with yourself after eating: "I just ate a 900 calorie dinner; do I really need to keep consuming food?" Avoid behaviors that are associated with food intake. If sitting on the couch watching TV encourages eating, go somewhere else in the house and read. And if you do watch television, indulge in abdominal crunches during the commercials, not Nestle Crunches.®

OUR PATRIOTIC DUTY

Okay, I will admit that this may be stretching things a little, but seriously, any source of motivation that keeps you on the healthy track is worth considering. Engaging in the habits of good health is not only advantageous to you and your family but also to your community and country. All insurance plans, including Medicare and Medicaid, involve distributing a pool of money to those who need it. If everyone consumed a daily breakfast of bacon, eggs, a six-pack of beer, and a few cigarettes, everyone would over-utilize health care, and the insurance model would not work. By doing your best to stay healthy, you are contributing to decreasing health care costs and keeping the nation's medical systems solvent.

Although the topic of medical care has obviously been greatly politicized of late, promotion of good health would appear to be something to which adherents to any political persuasion should subscribe. It is founded on a bedrock of personal responsibility, it lessens the transfer of wealth from people who take good care of themselves to those with self-destructive behaviors, and it allows the sustainability of national and state health programs that are vital to the well-being of our nation. Imagine how much less Medicare would cost if people simply adhered to the principles of this book. So, when you are asking not what your country can do for you, but what you can do for your country, allow me to give you an answer: perform your patriotic duty by eating a healthy diet and exercising regularly.

CONVINCING YOURSELF

We all have the capacity to change the way we look at ourselves and the world, and in some respects our perceptions are mutating each and every day. The strongest stimulus for reform that I see, as a doctor, is fear. Heart attacks, strokes, and cancer can turn burger-and-fries-for-lunch patients into vegetarians and two-pack-a-day people into fervent anti-smokers in a nanosecond. The point is that we *can* change, we do it all the time, and waiting for some disastrous event to instill terror into us does not make sense. There is no better moment than now to transform your thinking process and convince yourself that dietary restraint and unfettered exercise are pursuits worth building your life around. Maintaining good health is a lot like the way Hall of Famer

Yogi Berra amusingly described his life's passion: "Baseball is 90% mental; the other half is physical."

REREAD THIS BOOK

Everything in this book—from simple workouts, to energy expending activities of daily living, to easy dietary rules, to alterations in mindset—is geared to promote good health and IBW maintenance. So read it again if you begin to stray. You *can* do it!

Chapter 20

CHECKUPS

Many people are surprised to find out that I take medicine for high blood pressure (also known as hypertension). I guess they figure that anyone who exercises regularly, maintains his ideal body weight, adheres to a healthy diet, and watches his salt intake should not have hypertension. While these approaches certainly are part of nonpharmacologic blood pressure control, genetics can supersede everything. Therefore, you can be skinny as a rail and have hypertension. You can eat zero fat and have high cholesterol. And you can be thin and consume no sugar and have diabetes. The point is, I would never have known I have hypertension had I not had my blood pressure checked.

PRINCIPLE 19

Have yearly medical checkups.

Medical checkups need be neither extensive nor expensive, and if you're basically in good health, they don't even have to be yearly until you reach a certain age. Of course if there is a family history of hypertension, diabetes mellitus, high cholesterol, or breast or prostate cancer, you may need to be followed more regularly, but one checkup in your twenties, every two to four years in your thirties, every two years in your forties and every year after fifty is a reasonable schedule. Even if you have a high deductible in your health insurance or no insurance at all, you can have most of the recommended tests for the price of going to the movies a few times a month for a year. And periodic health fairs often will provide much of the checkup for free.

Here's what you should have checked:

1. Blood pressure.
2. Glucose (blood sugar).
3. Cholesterol—actually a lipid panel which also gives triglyceride and good (HDL) and bad (LDL) cholesterol levels.
4. Blood work for kidney tests.
5. Mammogram/breast exam/PAP smear to screen for breast and uterine cancers (ladies only—traditionally yearly PAP smears after age twenty-one or within three years of sexual activity have been advised, but recently the U.S. Preventative Services Task Force changed the recommendation to every three years; mammograms yearly after age forty unless family history).
6. Prostatic specific antigen (PSA) and digital prostate exam to look for prostate cancer—yearly starting at age fifty (and maybe stop after age seventy-five).
7. Consider a treadmill stress test if there is a strong family history of coronary artery disease at a young age.
8. Shingles (medical name, herpes zoster) vaccine at age sixty. The acute pain associated with shingles and, in some people, the accompanying chronic pain (post herpetic neuralgia) makes this vaccine well worth the money.
9. Abdominal ultrasound in men 65-75 who have smoked to screen for aortic aneurysm.
10. Colonoscopy. At age fifty then every ten years if no polyps are found. This is an expensive, invasive, and uncomfortable test, so, not surprisingly, it is the screening test that people most

often decline. The ability to allow early detection of colon cancer, or even remove polyps before they become cancerous, makes it an essential part of health screening.[1]

I had my first colonoscopy at age fifty, and although the prep was relatively unpleasant, the procedure itself was not too bad. I mostly slept through it. My uncle (by marriage) died of colon cancer after a miserable protracted illness punctuated by multiple surgeries. Some of his last words to me were, "Whatever you do, be sure to have your routine colonoscopies." I often relate this story to reluctant patients whom I'm trying to convince to have the procedure. Several of my patients have had early cancers that were easily cured, and they still thank me for talking them into having the colonoscopy.

Just because you feel fine does not mean that you are fine. Certain conditions, especially high blood pressure and high cholesterol, are notorious for not causing symptoms until it may be too late. You do not want to start treatment after you've had a stroke or heart attack but rather keep these from happening in the first place. So bring your body in for routine maintenance and checkups, and keep it looking new and running smoothly.

Chapter 21

MENTAL WORKOUT

I took Latin as my foreign language in high school because the conventional wisdom at the time was that it would be helpful if you wanted to pursue a career in medicine. Not true: it turns out Spanish would have been much more helpful. Latin was fun, though, and the best part was learning the Latin quotations from millennia past. My favorite was *mens sana in corpore sano*—"a sound mind in a sound body."

Stephen Hawking, the revered British theoretical physicist/cosmologist/author long afflicted with amytrophic lateral sclerosis, ALS, commonly known as Lou Gehrig's disease, has shown that one can be very productive with a great mind, even with tremendous physical disabilities, but the reverse is not true. If the mind goes, the body usually follows. In fact, a patient with brain death may still have a pulse and blood pressure but is considered to be dead nonetheless.

If you really want to appear younger than your stated age, you must not only be physically fit but must also have a sharp mind and a good mental attitude. Possible strategies to maintain mental fitness have been popularized as Alzheimer's disease has become more recognized. Though none of these strategies has been unequivocally proven, there is some evidence to support them, they make sense, and they certainly have little downside risk.

The main topics of much of this book, diet and exercise, may actually help to prevent the onset of dementia.[1] Proposed explanations include beneficial effects on blood pressure and cholesterol, thereby promoting better vascular health and improved blood flow to the brain. Whatever the mechanism, it has certainly been my experience that older patients who have led an active lifestyle infrequently develop dementia. Exercising the muscles likely helps the brain as well.

The most publicized dementia-busters have been brain exercises such as working crossword and Sudoku puzzles and playing cards. These activities keep the synapses firing, and one rarely encounters a demented bridge player. Reading newspapers or online news, keeping up on current events, and discussing them with others are excellent ways to exercise the mind.[2] Knowledge of world, national, entertainment, and sports news makes you appear younger, as you refuse to lose contact with the world around you.

I nearly always smile in approval when my eightyish patients tell me about working on their computers or using their smart phones. Technophobes of any age often miss out on opportunities for mental stimulation.

Intellectual pursuits may be one aspect of intact mental functioning. But in addition, mental health must be maintained. Now, doing crossword puzzles is one thing, but being able to keep calm and carry on in a tumultuous world is quite another, especially since we all face the ultimate train wreck at the end, whenever that will be.

Yet some people are able to maintain a positive, happy, optimistic outlook while others despair. Like most people, I've been happy, and I've been depressed, and undoubtedly, being happy is more fun. Many aspects of life are out of our control, but choosing happiness, though sometimes difficult, is certainly possible.

Over the years I have interacted with people during the most tragic and catastrophic times of their lives as they have dealt with personal illness or illness and death of loved ones. I have witnessed their coping mechanisms firsthand and distilled them, along with my personal observations during nearly six decades of life, into a list of recommendations for mental health maintenance.

1. Everything Zen. Adopt a Zen-like attitude. Take on life's setbacks with a calm acceptance, but maintain a resolve to do the best you can with the situation. Like everyone else, I am a work in progress, and I am still trying to conform to this piece of advice, especially related to the stress of my job. Anger and anxiety do not generally accomplish much but release stress hormones such as epinephrine (adrenalin) and others that raise pulse and blood pressure and may possibly cause vascular damage.

2. Live below your means. This was essentially the only financial recommendation that I gave to my children, and it is sound advice regardless of income. We obviously live in a very materialistic society, and probably there is some genetic predisposition to accumulating material goods, perhaps to show others that we are worthy potential mates. However, the things we buy rarely make us happy for long because our brains adapt to what we already possess. And soon we start to think about the next item we can buy. Humans tend to want things more than they like them once they have attained them.[3] Having money in the bank or in investments is much more comforting in the long run, and it is difficult to concentrate on a healthy lifestyle if you are consumed by financial worries.

3. Don't put off until tomorrow what you can do today. Enough said.

4. Stay married. Certainly, infidelity, physical abuse, and drug or alcohol addiction may be valid reasons for divorce, but many more couples separate for a variety of less irreconcilable causes.

If you ever want to achieve some degree of financial security, don't get divorced. Many if not most of my AYTSA patients have had long-term happy marriages. Of course, they may have good relationships because of personality traits that encourage AYTSA, not the other way around.

5. Understand life. To understand life you must understand that there is no understanding. The sooner you accept that bad things will inevitably happen to you, the more resilient you will become.

6. Rejoice in the small aspects of life. Whether it's the scent of a spring flower, the sight of your children playing their first violin or piano recitals, or the sense of accomplishment you derive from fulfilling your yearly goal, you must understand that life's rewards are more the actualization of the small things rather than major celebratory events.

7. Laugh. The absurdity of life is, if nothing else, entertaining. Learn to appreciate the humor and irony of the family, the business place, the political scene. Develop a self-deprecating sense of humor so you can show yourself and others that you don't take yourself too seriously.

8. Adjust your expectations. A useful equation to remember is $E - R = U$, or expectations minus reality equals unhappiness, a slight rewording of commentator Dennis Prager's equation from *Happiness is a Serious Problem*.[4] Having reasonable expectations—in other words, understanding that life is not always going to go your way—will diminish the gap between hopes and reality. According to a recent *60 Minutes* episode, Danish people are among the world's happiest, mainly because they adjust down their expectations.[5,6] My wife is of Danish ancestry, and one of my co-workers told me that she now understands the success of my long-term marriage.

9. Engage in prayer. For those disinclined to a religious thesis, meditation could substitute. However, my experiences have shown me that the people who are most effective in dealing with life's tragedies are those with a foundation rooted in faith, religion, and prayer.

10. Appreciate family and friends.

11. Have fun.

12. Travel. Nothing stimulates the mind and leads to introspection quite like seeing the way that other places and people do things. While not cheap, travel does not need to be terribly expensive in the Internet age (with online travel bureaus galore available) and with guide book authors like Rick Steves advising you.[7] And I would argue that travel is one of the most worthwhile ways ever invented to spend money.

13. Try to be the kind of person that your children can look up to. Be kind, hardworking, honest, faithful, and true to your word. If you're not, you won't be happy with yourself. And unhappy people don't appear younger.

Chapter 22

GENERAL APPEARANCE

As you can obviously discern, most of my emphasis on appearing younger has to do with regular exercise, ideal body weight maintenance, and attitude. External appearance also counts but may be less controllable than the issues that I've previously discussed. We are all confined within our genetic prisons, and certain aspects of our appearance, such as hair loss or familial tendencies toward wrinkles, may be more difficult to alter. But here are a few tips:

1. Wear a hat and sunscreen. Photo damage to skin from sunlight is a major contributing factor to wrinkling. If there is *any* planned sun exposure for more than a few minutes, these items are essential, and, in fact, many dermatologists recommend daily application of sunscreen for even those few minutes of solar exposure. Makeup now often has sunscreen added. Carrying a hat, sunscreen, and SPF 30 lip balm in your car will ensure that you will be protected in an unexpected situation. Don't forget to pay heed to often-neglected areas such as ears, lips, the back of the neck, and flip-flop-clad feet. And whatever you do, don't "work" on your tan either outside or in a tanning booth. Especially avoid facial exposure, which is inviting premature wrinkles, not to mention skin cancers.

2. Don't smoke. "Smoker's face" is an actual term in the medical literature.[1] Premature wrinkles. Don't do it.

3. Wear sunglasses. This may retard the development of wrinkles around your eyes and makes cataracts less likely. Furthermore, pterygiums, ugly growths on the sides of the eyeballs, occur more often with direct sun exposure.

4. Attire. If you maintain your ideal body weight, you can wear whatever you want. It's not like you are dressing to look young; it's that you do look young.

5. Floss. There are few aspects of your appearance that scream out, "I'm old," more than a set of dentures. Furthermore, dentures are a commentary on self-hygiene. The most common cause of the need for mass tooth extraction is periodontal or gum disease, which can be prevented by regular flossing, i.e., at least every single day. Additionally, there is growing evidence that flossing helps prevent the gum inflammation that can perhaps contribute to vascular events such as heart attacks and strokes.[2] Daily flossing may actually extend your life span. A high-speed electric toothbrush may help prevent gum disease as well but is no substitute for flossing.

Chapter 23

GETTING OLDER

Getting older. It's better than the alternative. It's not for wimps. The golden years aren't always so golden. We've all heard the clichés, which often have some validity. The universal truth about getting older is that it is inevitable. And to live life to its fullest, we must all adapt to the changes in our bodies that aging produces.

CHANGES ON THE OUTSIDE VS. INSIDE

From discussions with hundreds of patients in their eighties and beyond, I have learned that as we age we realize that our bodies have changed, but we still feel essentially the same inside. Wisdom increases with the years, no doubt. But basic personality traits, emotions, and personal guidelines for living life remain relatively constant. Reason, free will, and common sense, the triumvirate of human characteristics that lead to self-determination and self-discipline, remain intact. Therefore, we can continue to preserve control over much of our lives despite the aspects of aging that we cannot alter.

THE BATTLE TO MAINTAIN IBW

Aging conspires to make maintaining ideal body weight more difficult. Exercise is less comfortable. Joints ache. Lungs and muscles are less supportive of vigorous exercise. Recuperation from physical activity takes longer. Basal metabolic rates continue to slow. Our older selves require less food intake and more exercise at a time in our lives when most people do the opposite.

We must all accept aging, but we do not need to capitulate to it. The best advice is to stay active, and exercise the mind regardless of your age. Baseball legend Mickey Mantle famously observed, "If I knew I was going to live this long, I'd have taken better care of myself." You can plan for aging by accepting the changes but adjusting so they are as unobtrusive as possible. Staying active and maintaining your IBW are the best methods for combating the effects of age. As we've discussed, excess weight inordinately burdens joints, makes exercise more difficult, and starts the vicious cycle of sedentary living. If you wait until you're seventy years old and forty pounds overweight with aching knees and hips, your transformation to a vital, active senior will not be easy. It is sad indeed to hear stories from my patients who have fallen at home and are literally unable to get themselves up because of obesity, muscle atrophy, and deconditioning. Some of them have crawled around for hours, phones out of reach, until their plights were discovered. Maintaining IBW and keeping the upper body muscles strong by weight lifting could have prevented many of these episodes.

ACHES AND PAINS

Aches, pains, and injuries will certainly occur as you get older and may require taking time off from your usual exercise regimen. If that occurs, work out other muscle groups or shift to a different exercise that hurts less, e.g., stationary biking rather than walking, until the pain improves. Vary your daily routine so that, for example, you run every other day and weight lift every other day. This allows your muscles to recover and can diminish the likelihood of injury. Walking does not generally require such recovery and can be done daily. Weight lifting is important even for the elderly to strengthen muscles around joints, thereby better protecting them.[1]

Medications can help, but all have potential side effects. Acetaminophen is probably the safest. It has analgesic (pain relieving) properties but is not an anti-inflammatory agent. Liver toxicity is possible with an acute or chronic overdose, and you should limit it to 2.5 grams or less per day. In July 2011, maximum daily dose recommendations were changed by the makers of Tylenol from four grams to three,[2] but I would suggest 2.5 grams as a safety buffer. Daily heavy alcohol consumption may increase the likelihood of acetaminophen-induced liver damage. Also, acetaminophen is used in combination medications more than any other drug,[3] so read the labels to make certain you don't inadvertently take too much.[4]

NSAIDs (nonsteroidal anti-inflammatory drugs) such as aspirin, ibuprofen, and naproxen have both analgesic and anti-inflammatory properties and may work better if joints are red and swollen. These medications can irritate the stomach, damage the kidneys, and raise blood pressure, however, and should probably be avoided on a prolonged, everyday basis if possible. Certain NSAIDs may increase the likelihood of heart attacks, but evidence is far from clear. Prescription celecoxib (Celebrex) may offer less gastric complications but may still have the kidney and heart complications of other NSAIDs.[5]

Physical therapy, massage, and cold or hot packs obviously have a low incidence of side effects and may help alleviate the pain of an injured joint or muscle. If icing, freeze water in a paper cup and peel back the edge so you can comfortably hold it, or try placing a package of frozen peas on the injured area.

I find the most common reason that oldsters decrease their activity levels is because of pain related to degenerative arthritis in weight-bearing joints. It cannot be overemphasized that maintaining IBW is the best defense against the aches, pains, and debility of joint disease.

Impact

Low impact exercising may be necessary for some people with degenerative joint disease, also known as osteoarthritis. Walking, bicycling, swimming, water aerobics, or using a stair stepper may diminish joint pain as compared to higher impact endeavors. Those with back problems may find that recumbent bicycling is more comfortable. Walking, however, is the most universally applicable of exercises and should represent at least part of your regimen. If long walks seem too fatiguing, break up your walks to two or three shorter episodes per day. The more you can walk, the more you can do as the years progress, and most of the activities of daily living revolve around the ability to walk. A potential problem with low impact exercises such as swimming and bicycling is that they may be less likely to prevent osteoporosis.[6] Bone strengthening evidently requires some sort of weight-bearing stress application. Lifting weights, even light ones, should be a part of everyone's exercise program, and older people who sustain upper body strength will be better prepared to maintain their independence than those who do not.[7]

Balance

The less active you are, the worse your balance will become and vice versa. Balance is essential for older people to prevent falls and in turn one of the scourges of the elderly, hip fractures. Most hip fractures require surgery and hospitalization for four to seven days followed by physical therapy, often at a convalescent hospital for several weeks. It is a miserable injury that frequently takes a great toll on the elderly. Though often caused by tripping over various objects, it is sometimes simply the result of the loss of balance.

Most of the activities that I have encouraged throughout this book contribute to a better sense of balance. Physical therapy training should be sought if balance becomes a real problem with age and can be arranged through your doctor.

COMMON SENSE

As I write this, recent headlines in my newspaper report that a fifty-year-old body surfer was killed at the Wedge in Newport Beach. The Wedge is notorious for dangerous surf; waves refract off of a jetty and combine with incoming waves to produce huge peaks that break in a few feet of water. On a fifteen-foot day, the unfortunate man was dashed against the rock jetty and could not be saved. *What*, I wondered, *was a fifty-year-old doing out there on such a dangerous day?* Realize that limits will change as you age. Use common sense.

ACCIDENT PROOF YOUR HOUSE

I have seen many hundreds of patients with hip fractures, and I always ask how it happened. From stumbling over a pet to getting feet tangled in a hose to falling from a ladder putting up Christmas lights, I have heard all of the explanations. Some causes could simply not be prevented, but others certainly might have been had a little foresight been used.

The older you are, the more you should be aware of the potential to fall and fracture a hip. Pay attention to your balance during activities. Use great caution going up and down stairs; focus completely on every step. Adhere to a familiar route if you walk so that little bumps and potholes are known and therefore less threatening. Avoid sudden quick turns that can alter balance.

Eliminate clutter in the house, and never leave anything on the floor over which you could trip. Consider carpet rather than hard floors. Test small rugs for slipping potential. Always roll up hoses, and keep them out of the path of ambulation. Don't unnecessarily rearrange furniture. Look out for cement or asphalt that has shifted and produced a lip; consider marking these areas with red tape or paint if they are on your property.

Be very careful around pets that are congregating at your feet. Carry a small flashlight on your keychain for unexpected or unfamiliar dark areas. Watch out for speed bumps when walking in a parking lot. And if you're older than seventy-five, never ever get up on a ladder or stool; ask someone younger to do it for you.

ATTITUDE

Is age really relative? Are you truly only as old as you feel? Recent studies may actually support that a positive attitude about aging can be a self-fulfilling prophecy. Those who held negative stereotypes about the elderly at younger ages were less healthy when they became older than their counterparts who were more optimistic about aging.[8]

Although I do encounter the occasional patient who wonders aloud to me why God has not taken them yet, many older people I see are still having a blast. "I'm happier today than I've ever been," proclaims a ninety-one-year-old New York City woman in a quote from a *Wall Street Journal* article describing attitudes of oldsters.[9] Even in the elderly, if you think you can, you can, and if you think you can't, you're right.

CHECKUPS

Whereas a person in his twenties can often go several years without a checkup, those fifty and older should go at least every year or perhaps considerably more often depending on underlying health status. Sometimes subtle clues can identify a problem before it becomes a disaster. New or changing symptoms should be reported to your doctor promptly for the same reason. Refer back to Chapter 19, *Checkups*, for specific recommendations.

DELAYED GRATIFICATION VS. IMMEDIATE REWARD

Live in the now or prepare for the future? Many prescriptions for living are framed in this context as if they are mutually exclusive endeavors. The AYTSA lifestyle simultaneously allows for both. At any age, being physically fit and eating right will make you look better, feel better physically, feel better mentally and permit you to enjoy the present more fully. And as you maintain this lifestyle, whether you're turning fifty, sixty, seventy, or beyond, you will have spent your lifetime preparing for that moment. With a little luck and the proper lifestyle, your golden years can live up to their name.

Chapter 24

DIET BOOKS AND OTHER MYTHS

Popular culture is rife with dietary misperceptions, superstitions, and outright fabrications. To put it in nutritional terms, there is a lot of baloney out there. Surprisingly, even health care workers can share these misguided impressions, and I will admit that, during the research for this book, several of my long held beliefs were shattered by contemporary research. Here are some of my favorite diet and fitness myths:

MYTH #1: DIET BOOKS KEEP YOU SLIM

Going on a diet is one of America's great pastimes. People temporarily alter their eating patterns, lose a little weight, and go on their merry ways. Often they don't quite reach their target weights before they return to old habits, so, in fits and starts, their weight vs. time curve moves jaggedly upward. But getting to IBW and maintaining it is forever, so temporary weight reduction books aren't effective. Weight loss and weight maintenance are simply different points on the spectrum of what should be a diet for the rest of your life. Diet books work for only one scientific reason: calorie reduction. They often tout some novel approach to the intake and output principle by denying certain foods or promoting others. They are generally not suitable for the long term, and when the novelty wears off, the pounds come back on.

Some diets restrict certain carbohydrates, such as the Zone and South Beach. Others, like Atkins, eliminate all carbs and allow only fat and protein intake. French Women Don't Get Fat encourages you to indulge everything in moderation (not bad advice) but also in the magical powers of leek soup. The Sonoma Diet proposes a Mediterranean diet that includes (surprise!) wine. Sugar Busters says that sugar is taboo. Eat Right For Your Type is a diet based on your blood type. Other diets, like the cabbage soup diet, seem to exist only so that fad-diet bashers can ridicule them.

Again, these diets can lead to weight loss because they restrict calories. And some of them are actually suitable for the long term if you like the kind of food they promote. But what about designing your own healthy diet based on the MyPlate guidelines with your own preferences? Your own diet will be just as effective as the famous ones as long as you appropriately restrict calories for your needs.

A few other methods that deserve mention are Weight Watchers, which assigns a point system to limit calories, and NutriSystem, which delivers pre-made, calorie restrictive food. Both are very sensible methods that I would not discourage, but they still work for only one reason.

MYTH #2: FOODS WITH A HIGH GLYCEMIC INDEX SHOULD BE AVOIDED

Glycemic index refers to a ranking system of carbohydrates according to their tendency to immediately raise blood sugar after eating them. Low fiber starches and simple sugars such as white bread and sugar (the so-called white foods) raise blood sugar quickly and have a high glycemic index number. Carbohydrates with low numbers include whole grains and vegetables, which are more likely to result in slower release of sugar into the bloodstream. Immediate, high levels of blood sugar result in spikes of insulin secretion to drive the glucose from the bloodstream into cells, and the theory is that this stimulates more hunger and makes weight loss more difficult. There are only limited studies of this hypothesis, though, and nothing is conclusive. The general consensus by the American Dietetic Association is that avoiding high glycemic index foods does not aid in appetite suppression.[1] While ongoing investigation is in progress, it is reasonable to presume for the time being that a calorie is a calorie.

However … a frequently quoted article conducted a meta-analysis of a number of contradictory studies and concluded that there is an increased incidence of diabetes mellitus, coronary artery disease, and certain cancers with high glycemic index (GI) foods.[2] Whether this is statistical sleight of hand or genuine evidence is not clear. Even if the study's premise is true, one could argue that higher GI carbohydrates may not have been the culprit since the diets would have had less room for known healthy foods such as fruits, vegetables, fiber, whole grains, and soy protein. Common sense dictates that, while high GI carbohydrates may not interfere with IBW maintenance, they are, as designated in the MyPlate website, "empty calories," and you would be better served by filling up on fruits and vegetables and the rest of the healthy stuff.

Myth #3: Sugar Is Bad for You

This is more a half-truth but does involve controversy. When the term "sugar" is used, we generally mean:

a. sucrose or table sugar, a disaccharide composed of fructose bonded to glucose, or

b. high fructose corn syrup, which is sweeter than sucrose and is added to many foods to sweeten and/or stabilize them, or

c. honey, which is free fructose along with sucrose.

Other sugars of importance include:

d. lactose, which is milk sugar, and

e. glucose, which is the main sugar in the bloodstream but rarely eaten in its pure form.

Starch is actually many glucoses linked to one another. Salivary and intestinal wall enzymes cleave the molecular bonds yielding free glucose which is promptly absorbed through the intestine and into the bloodstream.[3] This is why some people consider low fiber starch, such as that in potatoes, to be equivalent to sugar. Fiber, which largely consists of non-digestible plant cell wall carbohydrates, delays glucose absorption. High fiber foods, such as whole grains and fruits and vegetables, can therefore be thought of as a time release form of glucose.

Sugar is bad for teeth, for diabetics, and perhaps for those with high triglyceride levels.[4] Nutritionaly, however, sugar is about like any other food; in prudent amounts it is fine, but if you eat too much, you'll get fat. It is a simple carbohydrate and has a high glycemic index. Sugar may cause more swings in insulin levels than complex carbohydrates, but, as above, there is no proof that this is bad for you. There is no evidence that sugar causes hyperactivity, diabetes, or hypoglycemia (low sugar levels).[5] Unless there is strong incentive (i.e., diabetes), it is unrealistic and unnecessary to eliminate sugar from your diet. However … if you find that sugar or other high glycemic-index carbohydrates make it more difficult to lose or maintain your weight, then by all means adjust your diet accordingly. Since sugar probably confers no nutritional benefits other than calories, eating more fruits and vegetables is a more healthy strategy.

To be fair, there are well-credentialed advocates of anti-sugar campaigns claiming that fructose is the major cause for obesity, hypertension, and diabetes. A recent commentary in the journal *Nature*, entitled, "The toxic truth about sugar," proposes that sugar should be regulated by the government like alcohol because it is so dangerous.[6] Is this the truth or just more nutritional bullsweet? The argument that the demon sugar, rather than overeating and under-exercising, is the cause for our obesity and cardiovascular epidemics seems a little far-fetched, and a scientific consensus is lacking.[7,8]

One of the rationales for sugar-bashing seems to be the fact that the metabolic pathway for fructose does make it more likely to be metabolized to fat via a process called de novo lipogenesis.[9,10] However, both fructose and sucrose are naturally present in fruits and vegetables, and lactose is one of the first foods we ever eat.[11] Furthermore, so-called fructophobia does not explain the Australian Paradox. A study of that country's residents from 1980-2003 showed a 16% reduction in sugar intake while the rate of obesity *tripled*.[12] Or the Twinkie Diet, whereby a Kansas State University nutrition professor lost twenty-seven pounds in ten weeks on a junk food diet containing predominantly Twinkies.[13] (Please, *do not try this at home*. This is not a safe diet, and he was only doing it to prove a point.) These examples are certainly more in accordance with the Intake and Output (I&O) Principle (see Chapter 4) than the sugar-toxicity theory. Again, there is little question that refined sucrose, high fructose corn syrup, and honey are not particularly good for you, but, in judicious amounts, do not appear to be harmful, either. And, in the unlikely case that you missed out on one of life's main lessons, too much of anything is generally bad for you.

Is sugar addictive? In his fascinating book, *The End of Overeating,* David Kessler presents evidence that certain "hyperpalatable" foods, those containing sugar, fat, and salt, are involved with higher dopamine release in the brain and rewire it to crave such foods.[14] This might be true for rats, but, as we have discussed, people are not only capable of self-regulation, they may be able to strengthen this human trait with continued use. So, sure, hyperpalatable foods taste great, but we don't have to eat them all the time.

MYTH #4: MEDICAL STUDIES REPORTED BY THE MEDIA ARE RELIABLE

Another half-truth. Some studies are well performed and the conclusions are valid but not all. The media is likely to report on a given study based on its sensationalism, however, not on its quality. The best way to test the effectiveness of a new medication (or diet) is to perform a randomized, double-blind, placebo-controlled trial (RDBPCT).[15] This involves randomly dividing participants into two equal-sized groups. Group A receives the medication while Group B gets placebo or sugar pills that look just like the medication. So there is no bias on either side, neither the participants nor the researchers know who gets which one (thus double-blind) during the study. After the study is completed, the effects of the medicine are assessed, and the difference between the two groups is subjected to statistical analysis. Only then is the code broken so that the researchers know which group received the real medication. The favorable (or unfavorable) effects of the medicine are thought to be reliable if they reach what is called statistical significance.

Many clinical studies are not done with a RDBPCT, which may diminish their reliability. And the supposed unbiased nature of RDBPCT studies themselves have been questioned of late.[16] The ultimate test of a scientific article's validity is reproducibility in subsequent studies. The frequent problem of non-reproducibility, even in the gold-standard peer-reviewed journals, has been referred to as "one of medicine's dirty secrets"[17] and is the subject of an entire recent issue of the journal *Science*.[18]

Even with a valid, reproducible RDBPCT, individual variation of human subjects means that some participants may not respond to the medicine despite the achievement of statistical significance. So, while a medicine could be found to be beneficial in a well-designed clinical trial, it may not be effective in an individual patient. Furthermore, the media often broadcasts a preliminary study as dictum when it may require considerable further investigation before it becomes an acceptable part of medical or nutritional therapy. We should always have some degree of caution when interpreting these studies; nothing is absolute.

MYTH #5: YOU SHOULD DRINK AT LEAST EIGHT GLASSES OF WATER PER DAY

Humans possess a sensitive thirst center in part of the brain called the hypothalamus, which responds to dehydration and tells the body to drink more water. The amount needed varies from person to person. So instead of targeting a certain number of glasses of water per day, we can simply rely upon our thirst to tell us it's time to drink water, barring some sort of brain injury. Whether or not the gastric distension that drinking excess water produces can decrease appetite is debatable, though some studies have shown a benefit.[19] There is some evidence that volume of a liquid, not caloric content, is the stronger determinant of satiety,[20] again emphasizing the inadvisability of drinking sugary beverages such as soda. As usual, common sense prevails, so if drinking water seems to curb your appetite, then go for it.

MYTH #6: EATING BEFORE BEDTIME PUTS ON MORE FAT THAN EATING EARLIER IN THE DAY

Review Principle 2 in Chapter 4 again. It's all intake and output of calories, and the time of day makes no difference.

MYTH #7: CERTAIN FAT BURNING FOODS HELP YOU LOSE WEIGHT

No elaboration is necessary. No such food exists.

Myth #8: You Must Do Sit-Ups to Have a Flat Abdomen

If you want to have six pack abs, then, yes, abdominal exercise to enlarge or hypertrophy the muscles is necessary. But losing fat has to do with the I&O principle—it will happen if output exceeds input regardless of what parts of the body you exercise.

Myth #9: Dairy Products Are Bad For You

Proponents of this view are fond of stating that milk is the perfect food … if you're a calf. And the dairy industry has no doubt influenced the USDA recommendations to include their products in MyPlate, the Food Pyramid, and the Basic Four food groups, a concern that should rightly raise skeptical eyebrows. Milkfat is certainly a calorically dense food; its high saturated fat content can contribute to the adverse consequences of high cholesterol, and it should be consumed sparingly. But … nonfat dairy products such as nonfat milk, yogurt, and cottage cheese can provide inexpensive, high protein, low calorie, satiating nutrition to a largely plant-based diet. Obviously, those with a dairy allergy or lactose intolerance may need to find non-dairy substitutes. Greek yogurt is lower in lactose, and smaller servings, e.g., four ounces, of milk may not cause problems in some lactose intolerant individuals.[21] And questionable claims of dairy's link to prostate and ovarian cancers will someday either be proven or dispelled. In the meantime, I contend that *nonfat* dairy products can be an important ingredient in the ideal-body-weight diet, and they are included in nearly every one of my meals.

Myth #10: Eggs Are Bad For You

This is more of a partial myth. The bad "ovo-reputation" is because an egg yolk contains approximately 200 milligrams of cholesterol, about two-thirds of the recommended daily limit. The good news is that at 75 calories, one egg has 6 grams of protein and 5 grams of fat but only about 1.5 grams of saturated fat. Evidence is mounting that intake of saturated fat may be more important than consuming cholesterol itself in the development of high cholesterol and cardiovascular disease.[22,24] So, let us review the good, the bad, and the extremely bad of dietary fat.

Dietary fat is derived from either plants (if unadulterated, generally good fat) or animals (in general, bad fat). Although there has been a trend toward lower fat diets over the past four decades, the type of fat is more important than the amount. Fat is not soluble in blood, so as it is absorbed from the intestines, it is assembled into protein covered units called lipoproteins that dissolve in blood and carry fat to the body's cells. There are five major classes of lipoproteins but the most important for our discussion are LDL and HDL. Low-density lipoproteins (LDL) carry cholesterol, and if levels are too high they can cause cholesterol plaque to develop on the inner arterial walls, including cerebral and coronary arteries, leading to heart attacks and strokes. This is the bad cholesterol. High-density lipoproteins (HDL) take cholesterol from the bloodstream, from LDL, and from artery walls to the liver where it can be excreted. High levels of HDL protect against arteriosclerosis, so this is the good cholesterol.[23]

Unsaturated fats, the good dietary fats, are plant derived, may have cholesterol-lowering properties, and exist in liquid form at room temperature. The two types are monounsaturated and polyunsaturated fats. The latter includes omega-3 fats, present in fish, flaxseed, walnuts, olive oil, and other components of a Mediterranean diet. They may decrease the incidence of coronary artery disease.

Saturated fats are the bad fats. They are mostly animal derived and not essential components of a diet because the body naturally makes saturated fat and cholesterol. Meat, seafood, poultry with skin, and milkfat are the primary sources. A few plant oils like coconut and palm oils, found in commercially baked goods, candies, and desserts, are saturated fats. And, interestingly, nuts, which are thought to perhaps confer cardioprotective effects, actually contain a few grams of saturated fat per one ounce serving. High saturated fat intake can increase LDL, the bad cholesterol.[21,24]

Trans fats are the extremely bad fats, and even small amounts may not only increase LDL but also decrease HDL. They are made by heating vegetable oils with hydrogen gas. Deep fried fast foods, bakery products, and packaged sweets are the major sources, but recent government interventions, such as labeling requirements, have lessened the prevalence of these fats.[25] The American Heart Association recommends intakes of less than 7% of daily calories as saturated fat and of trans fat, less than 1%.[21] Assuming a 2000 calorie diet, this would represent about 15 grams and 2 grams respectively. Fifteen grams of saturated fat is only a little more than a shot glass full of cream!

Studies have shown only a mild correlation between cholesterol intake and blood cholesterol levels. For certain individuals, however, blood cholesterol can decrease significantly on a low cholesterol diet. Who will and will not respond can only be determined by trying the low cholesterol diet. For many people, however, saturated fat intake may be more important than decreasing cholesterol consumption in maintaining low blood cholesterol levels.[22,24] Most cholesterol containing foods, though, are also high in saturated fats. Certain foods actually seem to decrease cholesterol. A recent study evaluated a diet containing a "portfolio" of cholesterol lowering foods including fiber, soy protein, nuts (both pea and tree), and legumes and found that it lowered cholesterol even more than did a low saturated fat diet.[26]

Which brings us back to the egg. Despite its high cholesterol content, it actually is low in saturated fat and therefore may not be as bad for you as was once thought.

MYTH #11: TO BECOME FAT YOU NEED TO EAT FAT

Definitely not true. Although fat does represent concentrated calories (see Chapter 4), a more accurate statement would be to become fat you need to eat *too much*. Excess carbohydrate calories can be stored as carbohydrates—for example, glycogen in liver and muscle—or as fat by a process called de novo lipogenesis. Furthermore, carbs may preferentially be used for immediate energy, thereby suppressing immediate fat metabolism and channeling it to fat stores.[27]

Again, the intake and output principle resurfaces. Despite the fact that percentages of caloric intake from fat decreased over the past thirty years, our obesity epidemic demonstrates that people have simply made up for lower fat by overeating carbohydrates. One 2006 study followed 49,000 women for eight years. Those who ate a low fat diet had the same incidence of heart attacks and strokes and maintained the same weight as those who did not.[28] And the *New England Journal of Medicine* article cited in Chapter 4 showed that calories, not components of a diet, are the determinants of weight regulation.[29] Certainly a low fat diet, especially low in saturated fats, makes sense and can be helpful with both weight loss and weight maintenance, but it's the total caloric balance that counts.

MYTH # 12: TAKE YOUR VITAMINS EVERY DAY

Futuristic predictions have often envisioned that everyone pops a tablet for breakfast that contains all the nutrients for an entire day. This magic pill is widely sought and is the theme of many diet books, even in the present day. Dietary supplements, including vitamins, minerals, and a multitude of other untested compounds are taken by millions of people every day with the hope that they provide better health.

Whereas pharmaceutical companies must show that medications are safe and effective in order to get Food and Drug Administration

(FDA) approval, dietary supplements are subject to a different, more lenient set of rules: the 1994 Dietary Supplement Health and Education Act. As you watch advertisements for Extenze® or Centrum Silver Women 50+®, it is useful to bear in mind the following points:

a. The burden is on the FDA to demonstrate that dietary supplements are harmful before they can intervene.

b. Supplement manufacturers do not need to inform the FDA or consumers about any data they have regarding the safety of the supplements.

c. Manufacturers are not required to substantiate the supposed benefits of their products.

d. Dietary supplement sales represent a $20 billion a year business.[30]

Based on these facts alone one should be highly skeptical of the claims made by the dietary supplement companies. The rules are permissive, the profits abundant, and the proof of effectiveness studies lacking. So how can you decide whether to take dietary supplements?

First of all, it is convenient to categorize dietary supplements into two groups: (1) vitamins/minerals, which everyone needs to ingest in one form or another, and (2) everything else, a group of compounds which are not essential but are taken for their alleged beneficial health effects. Modern nutritional science actually began with the recognition that certain vitamin deficiencies cause disease, such as scurvy (Vitamin C), rickets (Vitamin D), and beriberi (thiamine). There are thirteen vitamin groups and even more trace elements, which we all need but do not manufacture in our bodies, so we must ingest them.[31]

A balanced diet generally provides all of these vitamins and minerals so that most people do not require supplemental vitamin pills, exceptions being Vitamin B12 for those who eat no animal products at all, folic acid for women of childbearing age, and, if blood tests indicate deficiency, Vitamin B12 and Vitamin D in the elderly.[32] Regarding higher doses of Vitamins C and E for their antioxidant properties, the American Heart Association has concluded that "the scientific data does not justify the use of antioxidant supplements for cardiovascular disease risk reduction."[33] Furthermore, certain vitamins taken in higher than recommended doses can be toxic, and for some reason people often adopt the attitude that more is better when taking vitamins. A recent study concluded that even usual recommended doses were associated with increased mortality in older women.[34] Another consideration is cost, as supplements can vary from cheap, $3 to $4 per month, to fairly expensive, $50 monthly for individually wrapped vitamin packets. Even the most accepted of mineral supplements, calcium for osteoporosis prevention, is, according to the National Osteoporosis Foundation, indicated only when dietary calcium intake is not sufficient.[35] And a recent study indicating possible increased incidence of heart attacks with calcium use emphasizes that lack of benefit may not be the worst consequence of taking vitamin/mineral supplements.[36]

So what to do? As a registered dietitian colleague has opined, someone eating a healthy diet should not need to take vitamins. "But," she adds only half-jokingly, "most people don't eat healthy diets." Controversy abounds, and future scientific studies may provide clarity. In the meantime, I would recommend either no vitamin supplements or taking an inexpensive, generic one-a-day vitamin, assuming no actual vitamin deficiencies. Abiding by full disclosure, I take one vitamin tablet a day but certainly cannot argue with those who propose that if you want to increase your vitamin intake, eat more fruits and vegetables.[30]

The non-vitamin/mineral dietary supplements, which include amino acids and various botanical and non-herbal products, are a different story altogether. Unlike vitamins, MSM, Echinacea, St. John's Wort, and all the rest are not necessary for survival. And, as should be clear from the 1994 Dietary Supplement Health and Education Act, there is no burden of proof on their manufacturers to back up their claims of benefits or safety. Sadly, there is such a prevalent distrust of the pharmaceutical industry today that many people mistakenly believe that taking dietary supplements is somehow safer than FDA approved medications. For those wishing further reading material evaluating FDA approved medications as well as dietary supplements, I would refer you to what I consider the best medical journal in the world, *The Medical Letter On Drugs and Therapeutics*. While containing some medical jargon, it is concise, no more than four pages long, and written so that most anyone can understand it. I am reluctant to prescribe any medication that hasn't been vetted and approved by *The Medical Letter*.

I will admit that I know very reputable rheumatologists who recommend chondroitin-glucosamine for joint pains and cardiologists who prescribe coenzyme Q10 to patients who have muscle aches from statins. Overall, however, it violates common sense to put unproven, loosely regulated chemicals into your body. I neither take nor recommend non-vitamin/mineral dietary supplements.

MYTH #13: COLON CLEANSING REMOVES BODY TOXINS

This idea should be flushed down the toilet. Colon "cleansing" can be approached from above with oral preparations or below with colonic irrigation. Potential adverse consequences include bloating, diarrhea, cramping, flatulence, infections, electrolyte abnormalities, and colon perforation. If that doesn't scare you, how about the fact that there is absolutely no proven benefit to these procedures?[37] Furthermore, advocates of colon cleansing always refer to unnamed "toxins," the scientific basis for which is lacking. A much better and less expensive strategy for promoting intestinal health is simply to eat fruits, vegetables, and fiber.

MYTH #14: OBESE PEOPLE CANNOT BE HEALTHY

Obesity is associated with a greater incidence of high blood pressure, diabetes, and high cholesterol, and these maladies account for much of the increased health risks of the obese. On the other hand, an overweight patient who controls with medications his blood pressure, cholesterol, and glucose level could even be healthier than a thinner person who does not. In general, however, maintaining IBW is by far the healthiest choice.

MYTH #15: YOU CAN STAY FIT BY EXERCISING FOR THIRTY MINUTES THREE TIMES A WEEK

I know that I'm being repetitious here, but this important point deserves reemphasis. Never since *Homo sapiens* first roamed the earth have we sat around twenty-three and a half hours a day three days a week and twenty-four hours for the other four. That is, until now. To believe that we can spend 0.9% of our lives being active and hope to stay physically fit is engaging in magical thinking of the highest order. Pursuit of food and shelter necessitated exercise by our ancestors, so evolution hardwired a need to be active. Portions of all of our days are spent in certain obligatory activities, including eating, sleeping, working, and family matters. Exercise should be one of these requisites. At least an hour a day, not counting activities of daily living. Every day. And as you age and your basal metabolic rate slows, more. Your life depends on it.

Chapter 25

HOW TO DIE

You may think that this chapter is a rather morose way to end the book. But dying is a natural part of living, and this book is about living life the right way. Furthermore, it is an important subject that needs to be disseminated. You won't find this in *The South Beach Diet.*

The only absolute certain aspect of our lives is that we're going to die some day, and yet we rarely talk about or plan it. When asked, most people say that when the time comes, they would prefer to die in their sleep, quietly and painlessly. But this way of exiting is the exception, so planning a little bit to try to make sure you're comfortable when that day comes makes very good sense.

Unfortunately, too many people die in the intensive care unit (ICU) of a hospital, and they often don't quite understand what that's all about. The high technology treatment in the ICU can perform miracles and save lives. But if you are older than eighty-five or if you have a terminal illness such as severe heart or lung disease or cancer, you should perhaps not be in the ICU in the first place, let alone die there.

Treatment in the ICU involves life support measures that are tremendously uncomfortable. An ICU patient will often have tubes down the throat, in the neck, in the nose, in the bladder, and in the rectum. They gag and choke continuously, they are in pain and discomfort from not being able to move around, and they must deal with monotony and tedium for days or weeks on end. These treatments may be justified if there is a reasonable chance of saving a life. But if you are elderly or have a severe chronic illness, ICU treatment may only cause a prolonged, agonizing death.

It is difficult to discuss death and dying, even with family members. As a consequence, many terminal patients end up on life support systems in the ICU simply because they didn't make it clear that they did not want these measures in the first place. Most patients on life support cannot talk, have their arms and legs restrained, and are heavily sedated. They are incapable of making their wishes known, and so surrogate decision makers, usually family, make the determinations. However, the emotional maelstrom of a critical illness in a loved one often clouds the judgment of family members. Not infrequently, guilt and indecision reign, and terminal patients suffer through weeks or months of life support before they die.

I often tell patients or their families that if I'm fortunate enough to reach my mid eighties, there is absolutely no way that I want to be tortured with life support systems. Likewise, when it's my time to go, I do not want someone doing chest compressions (and breaking ribs) or administering electric shock to try to restart my heart when it stops. If I am elderly or terminally ill, allow me to die in peace and dignity … please. And if I'm in pain or having trouble breathing, I want to be given morphine to relieve my symptoms. I have seen many patients pass away peacefully this way, and no one should have to die in discomfort these days.

PRINCIPLE 20

If you so choose, spell it out to your family members—DNR, Do Not Resuscitate (also known as No Code Blue).

And to those family members of elderly or terminally ill people: I know it's difficult, but please discuss the DNR issue with them. Not only does this allow self-determination, but it helps to remove the emotional pressure and potential guilt of having to decide this matter for someone else.

And as long as I'm being brutally honest here, let me have a word with my fellow baby boomers. I encourage you not to suffer through futile care in the ICU when you become elderly or terminally ill, simply on a humanitarian basis. In addition, our large population means that we could bankrupt the system that will be paid for by our children and grandchildren if we all choose to be placed in the ICU before we die. It has been estimated that 40% of an average Medicare patient's expenditures are spent in the last month of life. That is simply a non-sustainable financial outlay with baby boomers on the cusp of Medicare age. So talk to parents about themselves but also to your children about you. Tell your children if you do not want heroic measures when you become elderly or terminal, and repeat the conversation in years to come. You will be doing them, and yourselves, a great favor.

And don't worry, I didn't end the book on this note. There is a final and more uplifting chapter.

Chapter 26

THE NUDGE

L ife is often punctuated by seemingly inconsequential events that end up having marked impacts on our lives, like the blind date that leads to a long-term marriage or the college lecture that launches someone on a chosen career. My recommendations regarding healthy living did not all appear at once. They are an accrual of a lifetime of personal experience and the practice of medicine. Had I not been watching the 1976 Olympics one Sunday, I might not have been motivated to start running. Had my brother not sent my son a home video of weight lifting techniques, I may never have done my initial bench press. Had a high school friend not extolled the virtues of vegetarianism, I would, perhaps, never have had my first meat-free dinner. Had I not witnessed so much suffering from potentially preventable diseases, I could have strayed from my philosophy of lifelong fitness. And had a thought not popped into my brain one day, I might never have written this book. In each case, it was just a little nudge, just a happenstance occurrence, that led to profound changes in my life for the better.

In conclusion, I hope that this book is your little nudge. I hope that it will make you look into the mirror and vow that it is time for a change. It is never too late to realize that you can appear *and be* younger than your stated age.

Principles Revisited

PRINCIPLE 1: *Pursuit of a healthy lifestyle requires a personal transformation.*

Healthy living is not like breathing; it does not happen automatically. The efforts required to be healthy necessitate incorporation into self-identity. A healthy person becomes not only what you are but also who you are.

PRINCIPLE 2: *It's all I&O, intake and output of calories.*

This is the reason that any weight loss or weight maintenance program works. It's not magic; it's just thermodynamics.

PRINCIPLE 3: *People tend to overestimate output and underestimate intake.*

The Milky Way-Mile principle is a good illustration. Be honest with yourself, and keep track with pencil and paper if necessary.

PRINCIPLE 4: *If your weight goes above 5% over your ideal body weight, do something now.*

Once you are at IBW, never leave it. You must declare war on even mild increases in your weight.

PRINCIPLE 5: *You must will yourself to overcome the moment of truth.*

Getting to that first step of a walk or run is the most difficult part. Just remember how good and proud you'll feel when you're done.

PRINCIPLE 6: *Exercise every day.*

We evolved to be active. Three times a week is just not going to cut it. Cradle to grave.

PRINCIPLE 7: *Keep it simple and keep it comfortable.*

The less complicated the workout, the better the adherence. And it needs to be comfortable enough to sustain for the long run.

PRINCIPLE 8: *Bring a cooler.*

Bringing your own healthy lunch not only saves money, it may even save your life.

PRINCIPLE 9: *Be a creature of habit with a low fat, low calorie breakfast and lunch.*

It works and allows conformity with the I&O Principle, even when assigning more caloric latitude to dinner.

PRINCIPLE 10: *Use low fat salad dressing.*

Every calorie counts. Read the labels and choose realistic portion sizes.

PRINCIPLE 11: *Wait twenty minutes after eating or snacking to eat any more.*

When your brain doesn't yet realize that your stomach is already full, it's amazing what twenty minutes can do.

PRINCIPLE 12: *Don't tempt yourself.*

Keep hyperpalatable foods out of the cupboard. And don't go grocery shopping when you're hungry.

PRINCIPLE 13: *Make eating out a special occasion.*

Eating restaurant food regularly is simply not compatible with weight loss, weight maintenance, or good health.

PRINCIPLE 14: *Don't sit on your rear end.*

We have substituted television and computer time for hunting and gathering with predictable results.

PRINCIPLE 15: *Take the stairs whenever possible.*

Every bit of caloric expenditure helps. Use your imagination.

PRINCIPLE 16: *Have a physical endurance goal each year.*

A physical endurance goal means months of forced training, and the good exercise habits seem to permeate the rest of the year.

PRINCIPLE 17: *Early to bed, early to rise, helps you maintain your ideal body size.*

Exercising early means you won't be too tired after work or forget or be distracted by the inevitable daytime demands.

PRINCIPLE 18: *One pound of fat = 3500 calories.*

Divide by seven and you get the 500 Calorie Rule. Any combination of reduced food intake and increased activity totaling 500 calories per day yields the reasonable and sustainable pace of one pound of weight loss per week.

PRINCIPLE 19: *Have yearly medical checkups.*

You may eat the right foods and exercise every day, but if you have untreated high blood pressure, diabetes, or high cholesterol, you still will not be healthy.

PRINCIPLE 20: *If you so choose, spell it out to your family members— DNR, Do Not Resuscitate (also known as No Code Blue).*

I know it's disturbing, but no one gets out alive, and it is an important topic to discuss with your family.

RECIPES

The following dinner recipes are a lot like the rest of the book: simple and straightforward. They are the meals that have sustained my family for the past thirty years but should be personalized to your specific tastes. The recipes are vegetarian, but adding skinless chicken or fish would certainly be in accordance with a health-conscious diet.

As stated in Chapter 12, a side dish of vegetables and a salad complete the meal. Don't forget that you could sabotage all your efforts by eating a calorie- and saturated fat-laden dessert.

The recipes presume a low-calorie, low-fat breakfast and lunch as discussed in Chapter 7, and the approximate nutritional components are included. Remember that limiting saturated fat to 7 percent or less of calorie intake (about 15 grams per day in a 2000-calorie diet) is considered a healthy strategy in preventing cardiovascular disease.

If additional protein is desired, sprinkle on soy protein nuggets available at health food stores. They are slightly crunchy and do not alter the taste of the entrée. One quarter-cup serving contains only 75 calories but adds 11 grams of protein.

To your health!

TOMATO AND BASIL PASTA

Makes 2 servings

1 14-oz. can diced tomatoes
4 oz. whole grain thin spaghetti
1 whole onion, thinly sliced
1 Tbs. olive oil
½ cup fresh basil, chopped
½ cup parmesan cheese, grated

In large frying pan sauté onion in oil for about 5 minutes. Add can of diced tomatoes. While sautéing onion, bring water to boil in large saucepan. Add spaghetti and boil for 6 minutes. With slotted spoon add the spaghetti to the tomato mixture in the frying pan. Add chopped basil and top with parmesan cheese.

Double recipe, refrigerate, and serve later in the week.

Per serving: 380 calories
         19 grams protein
         15 grams fat
         5 grams saturated fat

VEGETARIAN BURGER WITH ONIONS, TOFU, AND MUSHROOM SOUP

Makes 2 servings

2 original Gardenburgers®

1 can mushroom gravy

1 onion, chopped

1 Tbs. olive oil

3 oz. baked tofu (comes in 6-oz. package with flavors such as hickory)

Sauté onion in olive oil until soft, about 5 minutes in frying pan. Add garden burger and crumbled tofu and cook until slightly brown on both sides. Add can of mushroom soup and cook until hot.

Per serving: 288 calories

11 grams protein

16.5 grams fat

4.5 saturated fat

EGGS AND POTATO FRITTATA

Makes 2 servings

2 red potatoes, sliced thin (approximately 4 oz.)

½ cup chopped onion

2 whole eggs

4 egg whites

¼ cup whole milk

1 tsp. fresh thyme

½ cup parmesan cheese, grated

½ tsp. salt and pepper

Preheat oven to 350 degrees.

Sauté onion in medium oven-safe frying pan until transparent, about 5 minutes. While sautéing, boil sliced potatoes in a saucepan for about 3 minutes. Don't overcook because they will be too mushy when added to the egg mixture. Add potatoes to onions in pan and stir to mix. Mix eggs, egg whites, and milk together in a bowl and whisk with a fork or whisk. Add mixture to frying pan, then add thyme and salt and pepper. Add parmesan cheese on top. Put into oven and bake for about 15–20 minutes or until it rises a little on top and looks done.

Per serving: 345 calories

24 grams protein

20 grams fat

4.5 grams saturated fat

PERIOGIES WITH ONIONS AND CORN

Makes 3 servings

1 package frozen pierogies (1 lb. or 12 pierogies)

1 large onion, thinly sliced

1 cup frozen corn

1 Tbs. olive oil

½ cup parmesan cheese, grated

½ tsp. salt and pepper

Heat oil in large frying pan. Add thinly sliced onion, corn, salt, and pepper. Sauté until onion and corn are golden brown. While browning the onion and corn, heat a large pan of water to boiling. Drop pierogies in and boil gently (a very high boil may cause pierogies to come apart) for approximately 4 minutes. Place pierogies into frying pan with a slotted spoon. Stir pierogies in the onion mixture. Top with parmesan cheese and serve.

Per serving: (4 pierogies) 430 calories

        11.2 grams protein

        17.4 grams fat

        3.1 gram saturated fat

QUINOA WITH TOFU AND VEGETABLES

Makes 2 servings

½ cup quinoa

3 oz. baked tofu

½ cup onion

½ small chopped red pepper

½ small chopped green pepper

1 small zucchini, sliced (can substitute corn, broccoli, or carrots)

1 14-oz. can vegetable broth

1 Tbs. Italian seasonings

½ cup parmesan cheese, grated

Heat olive oil over medium heat in frying pan, add vegetables and seasoning, and sauté until tender, approximately 5 minutes. Add quinoa and tofu and sauté until lightly browned, about 3 minutes. Add vegetable broth. Turn down heat to low and cover for 15 to 20 minutes or until all liquid is absorbed. Serve hot with parmesan cheese sprinkled on top.

Per serving: 345 calories

23 grams protein

14 grams fat

6 grams saturated fat

VEGETARIAN CHILI

Makes 4 servings

2 cups kidney cooked beans	1 Tbs. chili powder
1 14-oz. can diced tomatoes	2 garlic cloves, chopped
1 14-oz. can vegetable broth	1 tsp. cumin
1 cup chopped red bell pepper	½ tsp. oregano
1 cup chopped onion	½ tsp. salt
1 seeded chopped jalapeno pepper	1 Tbs. olive oil

Sauté onions and bell pepper until soft, approximately 5 minutes. Add chopped garlic and spices. Add diced tomatoes, vegetable broth, and beans. Bring to boil and simmer for 30 minutes.

Per serving: 161 calories

10 grams protein

3.5 grams fat

0.5 saturated fat

Can add skinless chicken to garnish.

To prepare beans:

Bring a bag of beans (kidney, northern white, black, or pinto) to boil for 2 minutes. Remove from heat and discard water, then rinse beans. Repeat 2 more times. Beans will be ready for final boil.

This method supposedly removes some of the sugars from the beans that cause gas discomfort when eating beans. Canned beans haven't been cooked with this method and may cause more gas. You can freeze the unused cooked beans for another time.

BOBOLI PIZZA WITH SAUTÉED VEGETABLES

Makes 3 servings; 2 slices per serving

1 Boboli® thin crust pizza shell

½ cup sliced onion

½ cup sliced red pepper

½ cup sliced green pepper

6 asparagus stalks

½ cup pasta sauce

½ cup parmesan cheese, grated

½ cup low-fat mozzarella cheese, grated

1 Tbs. olive oil

Preheat oven to 350 degrees.

Sauté vegetables in olive oil in frying pan on medium heat until soft and partially caramelized, approximately 10–15 minutes. Spread pasta sauce on pizza, then spread vegetables and both cheeses. Bake in oven until cheese is melted, approximately 10–15 minutes.

Per serving (2 slices): 493 calories

24.5 grams protein

17.4 grams fat

7 grams saturated fat

WEIGHT LIFTING TECHNIQUES

I am certainly no body builder, but the following weight lifting techniques have served me well. They are basic and practical, and they have allowed me to participate in recreational physical activities without injuries. There are many books and willing gym trainers available to supplement these methods, but remember to keep it simple and keep it comfortable.

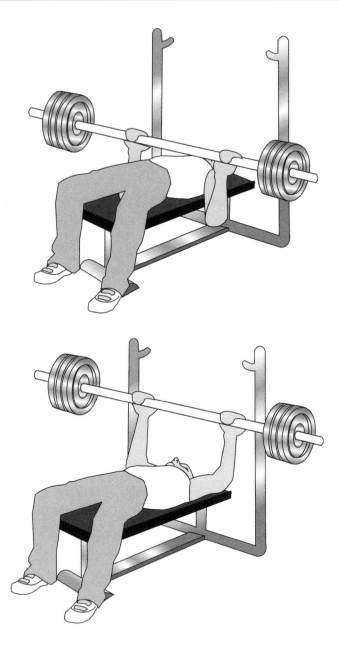

Bench Press: Four sets of ten repetitions.

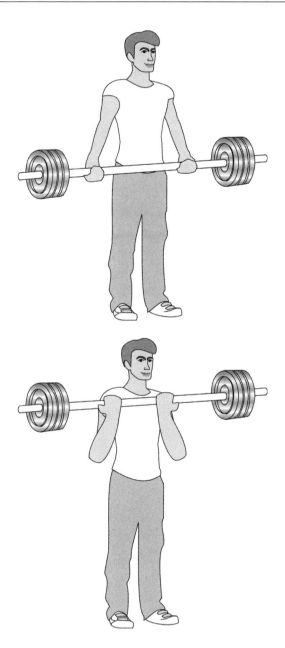

Curls: Four sets of ten repetitions.

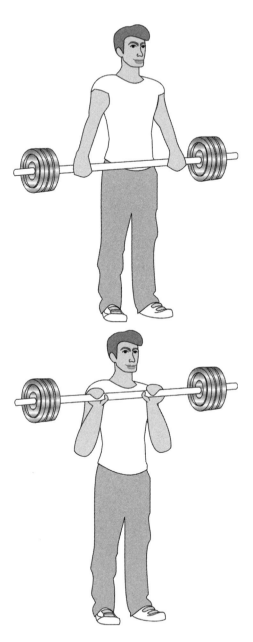

Reverse Curls: Four sets of ten repetitions.

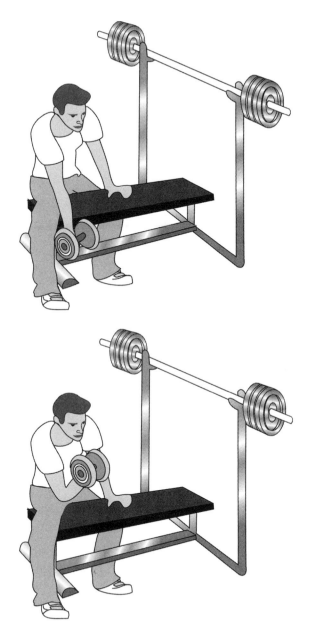

One-arm Sitting Curls: Four sets of ten repetitions, each arm.

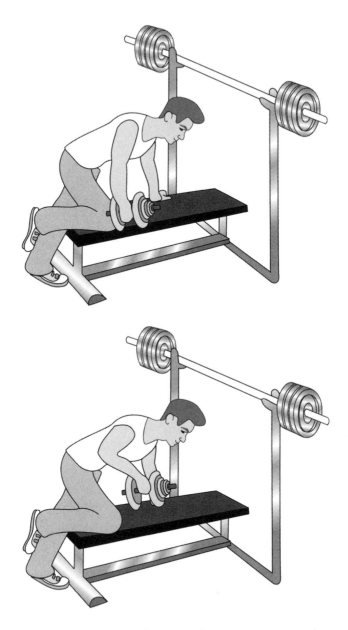

Chest Hoists: One set of twenty-five repetitions, each arm.

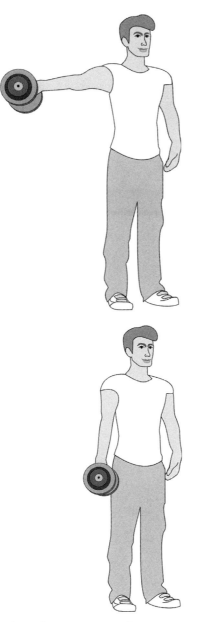

Side Lifts: Two sets of ten repetitions, each arm.

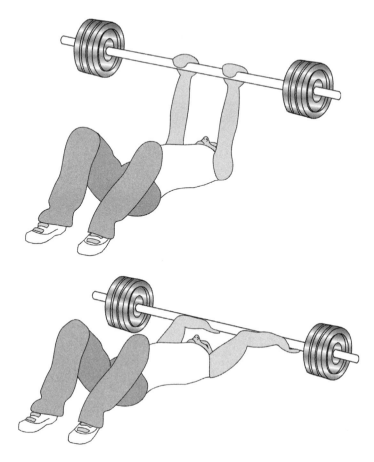

Behind-the-head Lifts: Four sets of ten repetitions.

Glossary of Terms and Abbreviations

Adipocyte: a fat cell.

Adipose tissue: fat tissue in the body.

Aerobic activity: activity that uses oxygen as part of the metabolic pathway (the Krebs cycle) that generates energy; usually submaximal exercise that can be continued for long periods; e.g., walking, jogging, and bicycling.

Alzheimer's disease: a common form of dementia usually beginning in late middle age, characterized by memory lapses, confusion, emotional instability, and progressive loss of mental ability.

Amino acids: carbon and nitrogen-containing molecules that link together to form proteins.

Anaerobic activity: activity that does not use oxygen as part of the metabolic pathway (glycolysis) that generates energy; usually maximal exercise that can be continued for short periods; e.g., weight lifting and sprinting.

Arteriosclerosis: narrowing of inside diameters of arteries due to deposition of cholesterol plaque; associated with strokes and heart attacks.

Atherosclerosis: see *Arteriosclerosis*.

AYTSA: Appears Younger Than Stated Age.

Basal Metabolic Rate (BMR): the energy that is utilized or burned from the metabolic processes that the body consumes at rest. Comprises about 70 percent of humans' total calorie expenditure.

Bell curve: in statistics a frequency curve that resembles the outline of a bell; average or mean is at the top of the curve.

BMI: see *Body Mass Index.*

BMR: see *Basal Metabolic Rate.*

Body Mass Index (BMI): an assessment of weight with respect to height; used to assess proper weight and similar to ideal body weight (IBW).

Caloric density: term used to express amount of calories present in a food with respect to its weight. Fat is more than twice as calorically dense than protein or carbohydrates.

Calorie: a unit of energy used to designate the energy-producing or, if not used immediately, the weight-gain potential of food. Also used to measure how much activity a certain physical activity requires.

Carbohydrate: one of three macronutrients (see *Fat* and *Protein*) representing a class of organic compound that includes sugars, starches, and cellulose and serves as a major energy source.

Cholesterol: a waxy substance produced by the body and present in all human cell membranes; high blood levels are associated with atherosclerosis.

Conditions that cause obesity: refers to under-exercising and overeating.

Coronary artery disease: narrowing of the arteries that supply the heart muscle with blood, usually due to cholesterol plaque. A predisposition to a myocardial infarction (commonly known as a heart attack).

Diabetes: a disease in which sugar and starch are not properly used by the body due to inadequate insulin production (type 1) or decreased sensitivity to insulin (type 2).

Dementia: severe impairment or loss of intellectual capacity and personality integration due to loss or damage to neurons in the brain.

Dietary fiber: the plant material that remains after digestion. May delay gastric emptying and promote satiety. Also may have a protective effect against heart disease and certain cancers.

Dietary supplements: products that contain a dietary ingredient taken in addition to the diet; includes vitamins, minerals, botanicals, herbs, among other compounds.

DNR: Do Not Resuscitate.

Ego depletion: term coined by psychologist Roy Baumeister to describe the fatigue of willpower with overuse.

Empty calories: term used in MyPlate to describe foods that contain fats and/or sugars but not much in the way of nutrients. Examples include pastries, sodas, and processed (not whole) grains.

Fat: one of three macronutrients (see *Carbohydrate* and *Protein*). An organic compound that is made up of carbon hydrogen and oxygen belonging to a group of substances called lipids. The most concentrated source of energy in foods.

Fat cell: any of various cells found in adipose tissue that are specialized for the storage of fat. Also called adipocyte.

Fructose: a sugar found in fruits, some vegetables, and honey. It is the sweetest sugar, and high-fructose corn syrup is used in many foods to sweeten or stabilize them.

GI: see *Glycemic index.*

Glucose: the main sugar in the bloodstream. The major food source for brain cells.

Glycemic index (GI): a ranking system of carbohydrates according to their tendency to immediately raise blood sugar and stimulate insulin release. Controversy exists as to whether foods with high glycemic index make weight loss more difficult.

Glycogen: a glucose polymer (glucose molecules linked to one another) that is used for glucose storage in animals.

HDL cholesterol: the good cholesterol that correlates with lower incidence of arteriosclerosis. HDL stands for high density lipoprotein.

Hyperplasia: abnormal increase in number of cells.

Hypertension: high blood pressure; a condition in adults normally described by a systolic pressure of greater than 140 mmHg or a diastolic pressure greater than 90 mmHg.

Hypertrophy: when cells increase in size and cause enlarged tissues and organs.

Hypothalamus: the part of the brain that controls several body functions, including appetite, water intake, temperature, and the release of many hormones.

IBW: see *Ideal Body Weight.*

Ideal Body Weight: a term describing the healthy amount that people should weigh based on height; derived from actuarial data and similar to body mass index (BMI).

I&O: Intake and Output; in this book the term is used to describe the intake and output of calories, an essential concept in weight loss and maintenance.

ICU: Intensive Care Unit where the sickest of hospital patients are treated.

Intake and Output: see *I&O.*

Internal organs: an organ or tissue that performs a specific function or group of functions within the body.

LDL cholesterol: the bad cholesterol that contributes to arteriosclerosis. LDL stands for low density lipoprotein.

Leptin: a protein hormone produced by fat cells that plays a role in regulating energy intake and energy expenditure.

Lipogenesis: the ability of the body to synthesize fat from other macronutrients.

Morbid obesity: a condition characterized by excessive body fat that correlates with a BMI over 40.

MyPlate: information from the USDA regarding healthy eating and lifestyles. Available online at choosemyplate.gov.

Nonpharmacologic control: control of a condition by engaging in measures other than taking medications.

NSAIDs: non-steroidal anti-inflammatory drugs, which include naproxen, aspirin, and ibuprofen; used to treat aches and pains.

Obesity: a condition characterized by excessive body fat that correlates with a BMI over 30.

Overweight: a condition characterized by excessive body fat that correlates with a BMI over 25.

Pedometer: a measuring instrument for recording the numbers of steps taken in walking.

Pharmacologic control: control of a condition by taking medicine.

Protein: one of three macronutrients (see *Fat* and *Carbohydrate*). Highly complex nitrogen containing compounds found in all animal and vegetable tissues. They are made up of amino acids and are essential for growth and repair in the body. Proteins are building blocks of enzymes, muscles, and some hormones.

Physiological: the way that organisms and their cells, tissues, and organs function.

Satiety: the feeling of fullness; absence of hunger.

Saturated fat: the "bad fat" usually derived from animal sources but also in palm and coconut oils. High intake of saturated fat may elevate LDL cholesterol and be associated with arteriosclerosis. Recommended not to exceed 7 percent of total calorie intake. Found in meat, seafood, poultry with skin, and milkfat.

Sedentary: characterized by a sitting position, meaning little activity.

Self-regulation: the term academic psychologists use in the scientific study of willpower and self-discipline.

Smoker's face: premature facial wrinkles caused by smoking.

Starch: a glucose polymer (glucose molecules linked to one another) that is used for glucose storage in plants.

Sucrose: table sugar; consists of a glucose linked to a fructose molecule.

Triglyceride: the chemical form in which most fat exists in food as well as in the body. Triglycerides are the body's storage form of fat and also circulate in the blood. High levels often appear with other well-known risk factors for heart disease.

Trans fat: the "extremely bad fats" made by heating vegetable oils with hydrogen gas. Intake may raise LDL and decrease HDL cholesterol and contribute to arteriosclerosis. Found in deep-fried foods, bakery products, and packaged sweets, though labeling requirements have decreased their prevalence lately.

Unsaturated fat: the "good fat," usually plant-derived; may have cholesterol-lowering properties, and usually exists in liquid form at room temperature.

Vegetarian: someone who eats no meat, poultry, or fish.

Vegan: a strict vegetarian who eats no animal or dairy products at all.

REFERENCES

CHAPTER 1

1. Khaw K-T, Wareham N, Welch A, Luben R, et al. Combined Impact of Health Behaviours and Mortality in Men and Women: The EPIC-Norfolk Prospective Population Study. *PLoS Med*. 2008; 5(1): e12.

2. Ornish D, Lin J, Daubenmier J, Weidner G, et al. Increased telomerase activity and comprehensive lifestyle changes: a pilot study. *The Lancet Oncology*. 2008; 9(11):1048-1057.

3. Sherertz EF, Hess SP. Stated Age. *N Engl J Med*. 1993; 329:281-282.

4. DeGowin EL, DeGowin RL. *Bedside Diagnostic Examination*. Third edition. New York: Macmillan Publishing Company, Inc., 1976.

CHAPTER 3

1. Fatstats: Obesity and Overweight. Centers for Disease Control and Prevention. April 2, 2009. www.cdc.gov.

2. Ford EJ, Bergmann MM, Kroger J, Schuebkiewitz A, et al. Healthy Living Is the Best Revenge: Findings From the European Prospective Investigation Into Cancer and Nutrition—Potsdam Study. *Arch Int Med*. 2009; 169(15):1355-1362.

3. Cryer PE. Hypoglycemia. In Fauci AS, Braunwlad E, Kasper DL, Hauser SL, Longo DL, Jameson JL, Loscalzo, eds. *Harrison's Principles of Internal Medicine*. 17th edition. New York: McGraw-Hill Medical. 2008. 2305.

4. Maclean, Norman. *Young Men and Fire*. Chicago: University of Chicago Press, 1992. xiii.*

CHAPTER 4

1. Zinn SL. Body Size and Habitus. In Walker HK, Hall WD, Hurst JW, editors. *Clinical Methods: The History, Physical, and Laboratory Examinations.* 3rd edition. Boston: Butterworths, 1990.

2. Kushner RF. Evaluation and Management of Obesity. In Fauci AS, Braunwlad E, Kasper DL, Hauser SL, Longo DL, Jameson JL, Loscalzo, eds. *Harrison's Principles of Internal Medicine.* 17th edition. New York: McGraw-Hill Medical. 2008. 469.

3. Flier JS, Mararos-Flier E. Biology of Obesity. In Fauci AS, Braunwlad E, Kasper DL, Hauser SL, Longo DL, Jameson JL, Loscalzo, eds. *Harrison's Principles of Internal Medicine.* 17th edition. New York: McGraw-Hill Medical. 2008. 463.

4. Kirby J for The American Dietetic Association. *Dieting for Dummies.* Hoboken, NJ: Wiley Publishing, Inc., 2009. 20-21.

5. Foster GD, Nonas CA, editors. *Managing Obesity: A Clinical Guide.* Chicago: American Dietetic Association, 2004. 7, 50.

6. *Merriam-Webster's Collegiate Dictionary.* Eleventh edition. Springfield, Massachusetts: Merriam-Webster, Incorporated, 2003.

7. Kirby J for The American Dietetic Association. *Dieting for Dummies.* Hoboken, NJ: Wiley Publishing, Inc., 2009. 29.

8. Calories burned. www.dietandfitness.com.

9. Kirby J for The American Dietetic Association. *Dieting for Dummies.* Hoboken, NJ: Wiley Publishing, Inc., 2009. 42.

10. Foster GD, Nonas CA, editors. *Managing Obesity: A Clinical Guide.* Chicago: American Dietetic Association, 2004. 98-99.

11. Spiro HM. *Clinical Gastroenterology.* Second edition. New York: Macmillan Publishing Co., Inc., 1977. 152

12. Sacks FM, Bray GA, Carey VJ, Smith SR, et al. Comparison of Weight-Loss Diets with Different Compositions of Fat, Protein, and Carbohydrates. *N Engl J Med.* 2009; 360(9):859-873.

13. Katan MB. Weight-Loss Diets for the Prevention and Treatment of Obesity. *N Engl J Med.* 2009; 360(9):923-925.

14. Flier JS, Mararos-Flier E. Biology of Obesity. In Fauci AS, Braunwlad E, Kasper DL, Hauser SL, Longo DL, Jameson JL, Loscalzo, eds. *Harrison's Principles of Internal Medicine.* 17th edition. New York: McGraw-Hill Medical. 2008. 464.

15. *Ibid.* 463-464.

16. *Ibid.* 467.

17. *Ibid.* 464.

18. Frary CD, Johnson RK. Energy. In Mahan LK, Escott-Stump S, editors. *Krause's Food, Nutrition, and Diet Therapy.* 11th edition. Philadelphia: WB Saunders Company, 2004. 24.

19. Kirby J for The American Dietetic Association. *Dieting for Dummies.* Hoboken, NJ: Wiley Publishing, Inc., 2009. 34-35.

20. Flier JS, Mararos-Flier E. Biology of Obesity. In Fauci AS, Braunwlad E, Kasper DL, Hauser SL, Longo DL, Jameson JL, Loscalzo, eds. *Harrison's Principles of Internal Medicine.* 17th edition. New York: McGraw-Hill Medical. 2008. 462.

21. Lehninger AL. *Biochemistry.* New York: Worth Publishers, Inc., 1970. 492, 513.

22. Olefsky JM. Obesity. In Isselbacher KJ, Braunwald E, Wilson JD, et al. *Harrison's Principles of Internal Medicine.* 13th edition. New York: McGraw-Hill Medical. 1994. 448.

23. Janz KF, Kwon S, Letuchy EM, Eichenberger Gilmore JM, et al. Sustained Effect of Early Physical Activity on Body Fat Mass in Older Children. *Am J Preventive Med.* 2009; 37(1):35-40.

24. Flier JS, Mararos-Flier E. Biology of Obesity. In Fauci AS, Braunwlad E, Kasper DL, Hauser SL, Longo DL, Jameson JL, Loscalzo, eds. *Harrison's Principles of Internal Medicine.* 17th edition. New York: McGraw-Hill Medical. 2008. 467-468.

25. Kershaw EE, Flier JS. Adipose Tissue as an Endocrine Organ. *J Clin Endocrinology & Metabolism.* 2004; 89(6):2548-2556.

26. Flier JS, Mararos-Flier E. Biology of Obesity. In Fauci AS, Braunwlad E, Kasper DL, Hauser SL, Longo DL, Jameson JL, Loscalzo, eds. *Harrison's Principles of Internal Medicine.* 17th edition. New York: McGraw-Hill Medical. 2008. 463.

27. Kirby J for The American Dietetic Association. *Dieting for Dummies.* Hoboken, NJ: Wiley Publishing, Inc., 2009. 34.

28. Foster GD, Nonas CA, editors. *Managing Obesity: A Clinical Guide.* Chicago: American Dietetic Association, 2004. 200.

CHAPTER 5

1. Khaw K-T, Wareham N, Welch A, Luben R, et al. Combined Impact of Health Behaviours and Mortality in Men and Women: The EPIC-Norfolk Prospective Population Study. *PLoS Med.* 2008; 5(1): e12.

2. Ford EJ, Bergmann MM, Kroger J, Schuebkiewitz A, et al. Healthy Living Is the Best Revenge: Findings From the European Prospective Investigation Into Cancer and Nutrition–Potsdam Study. *Arch Int Med.* 2009; 169(15):1355-1362.

CHAPTER 6

1. Fauci AS, Braunwlad E, Kasper DL, Hauser SL, Longo DL, Jameson JL, Loscalzo, eds. *Harrison's Principles of Internal Medicine.* 17th edition. New York: McGraw-Hill Medical. 2008. I-49.

2. Blumenthal JA, Babyak MA, Doraiswamy PM, Watkins L, et al. Exercise and Pharmacology in the Treatment of Major Depressive Disorder. *Psychosomatic Medicine.* 2007; 69:587-596.

3. Scarmeas N, Luchsinger JA, Schupf N, Brickman AM, et al. Physical Activity, Diet, and Risk of Alzheimer Disease. *JAMA.* 2009; 302(6):627-637.

4. Frary CD, Johnson RK. Energy. In Mahan LK, Escott-Stump S, editors. *Krause's Food, Nutrition, and Diet Therapy.* 11th edition. Philadelphia: WB Saunders Company, 2004. 24.

5. Foster GD, Nonas CA, editors. *Managing Obesity: A Clinical Guide.* Chicago: American Dietetic Association, 2004. 200.

6. Frary CD, Johnson RK. Energy. In Mahan LK, Escott-Stump S, editors. *Krause's Food, Nutrition, and Diet Therapy.* 11th edition. Philadelphia: WB Saunders Company, 2004. 23.

7. Foster GD, Nonas CA, editors. *Managing Obesity: A Clinical Guide.* Chicago: American Dietetic Association, 2004. 201.

8. Hall C, Figueroa A, Fernhall BO, Kanaley JA. Energy Expenditure of Walking and Running: Comparison with Prediction Equations. *Med Sci Sports Exerc.* 2004; 36(12):2128-2134.

9. Levine JA. Exercise: A Walk in the Park? *Mayo Clinic Proceedings.* 2007; 82(7):797-798.

10. Bassett DR, Schneider PL, Huntington GE. Physical Activity in an Old Order Amish Community. *Med Sci Sports Exerc.* 2004; 36(1):79-85.

11. Foster GD, Nonas CA, editors. *Managing Obesity: A Clinical Guide.* Chicago: American Dietetic Association, 2004. 201.

12. Chakravarty EF, Hubert HB, Lingala VB, Fries JF. Reduced Disability and Mortality Among Aging Runners: A 21 Year Longitudinal Study. *Arch Int Med.* 2008; 168(15):1638-1646.

13. Galloway J. *Galloway's Book on Running.* 2nd edition. Bolinas, CA: Shelter Publications, 2002. 81-87.

14. Ekkekakis P, Petruzzillo SJ. The Relationship Between Exercise Intensity and Affective Responses Demystified: To Crack the 40-Year-Old Nut, Replace the 40-Year-Old Nutcracker. *Ann Behav Med.* 2008; 35(2):136-149.

15. Galloway J. *Galloway's Book on Running.* 2nd edition. Bolinas, CA: Shelter Publications, 2002. 169.

16. Murphy J. What's Your Workout? These 3D Abs Are Part of the Job. *The Wall Street Journal.* Sept 1, 2009. D3.

17. Cloud J. Why Exercise Won't Make You Thin. *TIME.* Aug 17, 2009. 42-47.

CHAPTER 7

1. Foster GD, Nonas CA, editors. *Managing Obesity: A Clinical Guide.* Chicago: American Dietetic Association, 2004. 210

2. Rinzler CA, Graf MW, Fischer L, Kirby J, et al. *Calorie Counting for Dummies.* Hoboken, NJ: Wiley Publishing, Inc., 2009.

3. Kirby J for The American Dietetic Association. *Dieting for Dummies.* Hoboken, NJ: Wiley Publishing, Inc., 2009. 51.

CHAPTER 8

1. Sinha R, Cross AJ, Graubard BI, Leitzman MF, et al. Meat Intake and Mortality. *Arch Intern Med.* 2009; 169(6):562-571.

2. Pan A, Sun Q, Bernstein AM, et al. Red Meat Consumption and Mortality: Results From 2 Prospective Cohort Studies. *Arch Intern Med.* Published online March 12, 2012. doi:10.1001/archinternmed.2011.2287.

3. World Hunger as a Reason for a Vegetarian Diet. www.vegetarian-society.org.

4. Pimental D, Westra L, Noss RF, editors. *Ecological Integrity: Integrating Environment, Conservation, and Health.* Washington, DC: Island Press, 2000. 121-137.

5. Ornish D. Holy Cow! What's Good For You Is Good For Our Planet: Comment on "Red Meat Consumption and Mortality." *Arch Intern Med.* Published online March 12, 2012. doi:10.1001/archinternmed.2012.174.

CHAPTER 9

1. Guthrie HA. *Introductory Nutrition.* 2nd edition. Saint Louis: The C.V. Mosby Company, 1971.

2. Graham DJ, Jeffrey RW. Location, Location, Location: Eye-Tracking Evidence that Consumers Preferentially View Prominently Positioned Nutrition Information. *Journal of the American Dietetic Association.* 2011; 111(11):1704-1711.

3. Weil A. MyPlate USDA Nutrition Guide Has Its Cracks. *Huffpost Healthy Living,* www.huffingtonpost.com, 6/3/11.

4. Grundy SM. Nutrition in the Management of Disorders of Serum Lipids and Lipoproteins. In Shils ME, Shike M, Ross AC, et al, editors. *Modern Nutrition in Health and Disease.* Tenth Edition. Philadelphia: Lippincott Williams & Wilkins, 2006. 1083.

5. Willet WC and Ludwig DS. The 2010 Dietary Guidelines–The Best Recipe for Health? *N Engl J Med.* 2011; 365(17):1563-1565.

6. Ballantyne CM, O'Keefe, Jr. JH, Gotto, Jr. AM. *Dyslipidemia & Atherosclerosis Essentials.* Fourth Edition. Boston: Jones and Bartlett Publishers, 2009. 64

CHAPTER 10

1. Ballantyne CM, O'Keefe, Jr. JH, Gotto, Jr. AM. *Dyslipidemia & Atherosclerosis Essentials.* Fourth Edition. Boston: Jones and Bartlett Publishers, 2009. 124.

2. Schuckit MA. Alcohol and Alcoholism. In Fauci AS, Braunwlad E, Kasper DL, Hauser SL, Longo DL, Jameson JL, Loscalzo, eds. *Harrison's Principles of Internal Medicine.* 17ᵗʰ edition. New York: McGraw-Hill Medical. 2008.

CHAPTER 11

1. Model D. Smoker's face: an underrated clinical sign? *Br Med J.* 1985; 291:1760-1762.

CHAPTER 12

1. Urban LE, McCrory MA, Dallal GE, et al. Accuracy of Stated Energy Contents of Restaurant Foods. *JAMA.* 2011; 306(3):287-293.

CHAPTER 14

1. Levine JA, Lanningham-Foster LM, McCraday SK, et al. Interindividual Variation in Posture Allocation: Possible Role in Human Obesity. *Science.* 2005:307(5709):584-586.

2. Bravata DM, Smith-Spangler C, Sundaram V, Gienger AL, et al. Using Pedometers to Increase Physical Activity and Improve Health. *JAMA.* 2007; 298(19):2296-2304.

3. Foster GD, Nonas CA, editors. *Managing Obesity: A Clinical Guide.* Chicago: American Dietetic Association, 2004. 125.

4. Shah S, O'Byrne M, Wilson M, Wilson T. Elevators or stairs? *Canadian Medical Association Journal.* 2011; 183(18):E1353-E1355.

5. Foster GD, Nonas CA, editors. *Managing Obesity: A Clinical Guide.* Chicago: American Dietetic Association, 2004. 132.

CHAPTER 15

1. Light RW. Clinical Pulmonary Function Testing, Exercise Testing, and Disability Evaluation. In George RB, Light RL, Matthay MA, Matthay RA, editors. *Chest Medicine: Essentials of Pulmonary and Critical Care*

Medicine. 5th edition. Philadelphia: Lippincott Williams & Wilkins, 2005. 104.

2. Hill DW, Cureton KJ, Collins MA. Circadian Specificity in Exercise Training. *Ergonomics.* 1989; 32(1):79-92.

3. Light RW. Clinical Pulmonary Function Testing, Exercise Testing, and Disability Evaluation. In George RB, Light RL, Matthay MA, Matthay RA, editors. *Chest Medicine: Essentials of Pulmonary and Critical Care Medicine.* 5th edition. Philadelphia: Lippincott Williams & Wilkins, 2005. 104.

4. Deutsch, R. *One Best Hike: Yosemite's Half Dome.* Berkeley, CA: Wilderness Press, 2007.

CHAPTER 16

1. Czeisler CA, Winkelman JW, Richardson GS. Sleep Disorders. In Fauci AS, Braunwlad E, Kasper DL, Hauser SL, Longo DL, Jameson JL, Loscalzo, eds. *Harrison's Principles of Internal Medicine.* 17th edition. New York: McGraw-Hill Medical. 2008. 173.

2. Morgenthaler TI, Lee-Chiong T, Alessi C, Friedman L, et al. Practice Parameters for the Clinical Evaluation of Circadian Rhythm Sleep Disorders. *Sleep.* 2007; 30(11):1445-1459.

3. Martin L, Doggart AL, Whyte GP. Comparison of physiological responses to morning and evening submaximal running. *Journal of Sports Sciences.* 2001; 19:969-976.

4. Dalton B, McNaughton L, Davoren B. Circadian Rhythms Have No Effect on Cycling Performance. *Int J Sports Med.* 1997; 18:538-542.

5. Fell JS. For best exercise, don't be lonely or late: Activities done in groups and early in the day seem to show the best success rates. *Los Angeles Times.* April 04, 2011.

6. Hill DW, Cureton KJ, Collins MA. Circadian Specificity in Exercise Training. *Ergonomics.* 1989;32(1):70-82.

7. Wertz AT, Ronda JM, Czeisler CA, Wright KP. Research Letters: Effects of Sleep Inertia on Cognition. *JAMA.* 2006; 295(2):163-164.

8. Baumeister RF, Tierney J. *Willpower: Rediscovering the Greatest Human Strength.* New York: The Penguin Press, 2011. 22-39.

CHAPTER 17

1. Katan MB. Weight-Loss Diets for the Prevention and Treatment of Obesity. *N Engl J Med.* 2009; 360(9):923-925.

2. Foster GD, Nonas CA, editors. *Managing Obesity: A Clinical Guide.* Chicago: American Dietetic Association, 2004. 199.

3. Weinsier RL, Hunter GR, Desmond RA, Byrne NM, et al. Free-living Activity Energy Expenditure in Women Successful and Unsuccessful at Maintaining a Normal Body Weight. *Am J Clin Nutrition.* 2002; 75(3):499-504.

4. Wing RR, Phelan S. Long-term weight loss maintenance. *Am J Clin Nutrition.* 2005; 82(1):222S-225S.

5. Foster GD, Nonas CA, editors. *Managing Obesity: A Clinical Guide.* Chicago: American Dietetic Association, 2004. 199-200.

6. Malik VS, Schulze MB, Hu FB. Intake of Sugar-sweetened Beverages and Weight Gain: A Systematic Review. *Am J Clin Nutrition.* 2006; 84(2):274-288.

7. Baumeister RF, Vohs KD, editors. *Handbook of Self-Regulation: Research, Theory, and Applications.* New York: The Guilford Press, 2004. 84-98.

8. Baumeister RF. *The Cultural Animal: Nature, Meaning, and Social Life.* Oxford: Oxford University Press, 2004. 310-315.

CHAPTER 18

1. Bravata DM, Smith-Spangler C, Sundaram V, Gienger AL, et al. Using Pedometers to Increase Physical Activity and Improve Health. *JAMA.* 2007; 298(19):2296-2304.

CHAPTER 19

1. Foster GD, Nonas CA, editors. *Managing Obesity: A Clinical Guide.* Chicago: American Dietetic Association, 2004. 202.

2. Levitin DJ. *This is Your Brain on Music: The Science of a Human Obsession.* New York: Plume, 2006.

3. Park A. iPod Safety: Preventing Hearing Loss in Teens. *Time.com.* Feb 21, 2009.

4. Cloud J. Why Exercise Won't Make You Thin. *TIME.* Aug 17, 2009. 42-47.

5. Griffith DE, Hardeman JL, Zhang Y, Wallace RJ, Mazurek GH. Tuberculosis Outbreak Among Healthcare Workers at a Community Hospital. *Am J Respir Crit Care Med.* 1995; 152:808-811.

6. Baumeister RF, Vohs KD, editors. *Handbook of Self-Regulation: Research, Theory, and Applications.* New York: The Guilford Press, 2004. 84-98.

7. Baumeister RF. *The Cultural Animal: Nature, Meaning, and Social Life.* Oxford: Oxford University Press, 2004. 310-315.

8. Schneeman BO. Gastrointestinal physiology and functions. *British Journal of Nutrition.* 2002; 88 Suppl. 2:S159-S163.

9. Hellmich N. Apple a day keeps the calories at bay. *USA Today.* 10-24-07.

10. Graber C. Water Before Meals Means Fewer Calories Consumed. *Scientific American.* 8-24-10.

CHAPTER 20

1. Martin GJ. Screening and Prevention of Disease. In Fauci AS, Braunwlad E, Kasper DL, Hauser SL, Longo DL, Jameson JL, Loscalzo, eds. *Harrison's Principles of Internal Medicine.* 17th edition. New York: McGraw-Hill Medical. 2008. 24-26.

CHAPTER 21

1. Scarmeas N, Luchsinger JA, Schupf N, Brickman AM, et al. Physical Activity, Diet, and Risk of Alzheimer Disease. *JAMA.* 2009; 302(6):627-637.

2. Rice E. Exercise Your Brain to Prevent Memory Loss. *Newsblog. mayoclinic.org.* Feb 9, 2009.

3. Nettle D. *Happiness: The Science Behind Your Smile.* Oxford: Oxford University Press, 2005. 115-140.

4. Prager, D. *Happiness is a Serious Problem.* New York: HarperCollins, 1998.

5. 60 Minutes. The Happiest Place on Earth Is ... Feb 17, 2008.

6. Christensen K, Herskind AM, Vaupel JW. Why Danes Are Smug. *BMJ.* 2006; 333:1289-1291.

7. Steves R. *Rick Steves' Europe Through the Back Door 2012.* Berkeley: Avalon Travel Publishing, 2011.

CHAPTER 22

1. Model D. Smoker's face: an underrated clinical sign? *Br Med J.* 1985; 291:1760-1762.

2. Durso SC. Oral Manifestations of Disease. In Fauci AS, Braunwlad E, Kasper DL, Hauser SL, Longo DL, Jameson JL, Loscalzo, eds. *Harrison's Principles of Internal Medicine.* 17th edition. New York: McGraw-Hill Medical 2008. 214-215.

CHAPTER 23

1. Questions and Answers About Arthritis and Rheumatic Diseases. National Institute of Arthritis and Musculoskeletal and Skin Disorders. www.niams.nih.gov, September, 2011.

2. www.getreliefresponsibly.com.

3. Acetaminophen Safety–Déjà vu. *The Medical Letter On Drugs and Therapeutics.* 2009; 51(1316):53.

4. King JP, Davis TC, Bailey SC, et al. Developing Consumer-Centered, Nonprescription Drug Labeling: A Study in Acetaminophen. *American Journal of Preventive Medicine.* 2011; 40(6):593-598.

5. Drugs for Pain. *Treatment Guidelines from The Medical Letter.* 2004; 2(23):47-54.

6. Smathers AM, Bemben MG, Bemben DA. Bone density comparisons in male competitive road cyclists and untrained controls. *Med Sci Sports Exerc.* 2009; 41(2):290-296.

7. Peterson MD, Gordon PM. Resistance Exercise for the Aging Adult: Clinical Implications and Prescription Guidelines. *Am J Med.* 2011; 124(3):194-198.

8. Levy BR, Zonderman AB, Slade MD, et al. Age Stereotypes Held Earlier in Life Predict Cardiovascular Events in Later Life. *Psychological Science.* 2009; 20(3):296-298.

9. Beck M. Health Matters: Starting to Feel Older? New Studies Show Attitude Can Be Critical. *The Wall Street Journal*, October 17-18, 2009.

CHAPTER 24

1. Duyff RL. *American Dietetic Association Complete Food and Nutrition Guide*, 3rd edition. Hoboken, NJ: John Wiley and Sons, 2006. 116.

2. Barclay AW, Petrocz P, McMillan-Price J, et al. Glycemic Index, Glycemic Load, and Chronic Disease Risk—A Meta-Analysis of Observational Studies. *Am J Clin Nutr.* 2008; 87(3):627-637.

3. Ettinger S. Macronutrients: Carbohydrates, Proteins and Lipids. In Mahan LK, Escott-Stump S, editors. *Krause's Food, Nutrition, and Diet Therapy.* 11th edition. Philadelphia: WB Saunders Company, 2004. 41-44.

4. Ballantyne CM, O'Keefe, Jr. JH, Gotto, Jr. AM. *Dyslipidemia & Atherosclerosis Essentials.* Fourth Edition. Boston: Jones and Bartlett Publishers, 2009. 63.

5. Duyff RL. *American Dietetic Association Complete Food and Nutrition Guide*, 3rd edition. Hoboken, NJ: John Wiley and Sons, 2006. 112.

6. Lustig RH, Schmidt LA, Brindis CD. The toxic truth about sugar. *Nature.* 2012; 482:27-29.

7. Katz D. Sugar *Isn't* Evil: A Rebuttal. *The Huffington Post.* 4-18-11.

8. Sharma AM. Why Banning Sugar Will Not Solve Obesity. 2-6-12. www.drsharma.ca

9. Lustig RH. Fructose: Metabolic, Hedonic, and Societal Parallels with Ethanol. J Am Diet Assoc. 2010; 110(9):1307-1321.

10. Keim NL, Levin RJ, Havel PJ. Carbohydrates. In Shils ME, Shike M, Ross AC, et al, editors. *Modern Nutrition in Health and Disease.* Tenth Edition. Philadelphia: Lippincott Williams & Wilkins, 2006. 74-75.

11. Ettinger S. Macronutrients: Carbohydrates, Proteins and Lipids. In Mahan LK, Escott-Stump S, editors. *Krause's Food, Nutrition, and Diet Therapy.* 11th edition. Philadelphia: WB Saunders Company, 2004. 41-43

12. Barclay AW, Brand-Miller J. The Australian Paradox: A Substantial Decline in Sugars Intake over the Same Timeframe that Overweight and Obesity Have Increased. *Nutrients.* 2011; 3:491-504.

13. Katz D. "Twinkie Diet": A Physician's Take on What Really Happens. *The Huffington Post.* 11-13-10.

14. Kessler DA. *The End of Overeating.* New York: Rodale, 2009.

15. Meldrum M. A Brief History of the Randomized Controlled Trial From Oranges to the Gold Standard. *Hematol Oncol Clin North Am.* 2000; Aug; 14(4):745-760.

16. Kaptchuk TJ. The double blind, randomized, placebo-controlled trial: gold standard or golden calf? *J Clin Epidemiol.* 2001; 54(6): 541-549.

17. Naik G. Scientists' Elusive Goal: Reproducing Study Results. *The Wall Street Journal*, December 2, 2011.

18. Jasny BR, Chin G, Chong L, et al. Introduction: Again, and Again, and Again ... *Science.* 2011; 334(6060):1225.

19. Graber C. Water Before Meals Means Fewer Calories Consumed. *Scientific American.* 8-24-10.

20. Bell EA, Roe LS, Rolls BJ. Sensory-specific satiety is affected more by volume than by energy content of a liquid food. *Physiology and Behavior.* 2003; 78:593-600.

21. www.choosemyplate.gov.

22. Lichtenstein AH, Appel LJ, Brands M, et al. Diet and Lifestyle Recommendations Revision 2006: A Scientific Statement From the American Heart Association Nutrition Committee. *Circulation.* 2006; 114:82-96.

23. Rader DJ, Hobbs HH. Disorders of Lipoprotein Metabolism. In Fauci AS, Braunwlad E, Kasper DL, Hauser SL, Longo DL, Jameson JL, Loscalzo, eds. *Harrison's Principles of Internal Medicine.* 17th edition. New York: McGraw-Hill Medical 2008. 2416-2418.

24. Jones PJH, Kubrow S. Lipids, Sterols, and Their Metabolites. In Shils ME, Shike M, Ross AC, et al, editors. *Modern Nutrition in Health and Disease.* Tenth Edition. Philadelphia: Lippincott Williams & Wilkins, 2006. 99-103.

25. Reducing Intake of Trans Fatty Acids. *The Medical Letter.* 2007; 49(1267):65-66.

26. Jenkins DJA, Jones PJH, Lamarche B, et al. Effects of a Dietary Portfolio of Cholesterol-Lowering Foods Given at 2 Levels of Intensity of Dietary Advice on Serum Lipids in Hyperlipidemia. *JAMA.* 2011; 306(8):831-839.

27. Hellerstein MK. No common energy currency: de novo lipogenesis as the road less traveled. *Am J Clin Nutr.* 2001; 74:707-708.

28. Howard BV, Van Horn L, Hsai J, et al. Low-fat dietary pattern and risk of cardiovascular disease: the Women's Health Initiative Randomized Controlled Dietary Modification Trial. *JAMA.* 2006; 295(6):655-666.

29. Sacks FM, Bray GA, Carey VJ, Smith SR, et al. Comparison of Weight-Loss Diets with Different Compositions of Fat, Protein, and Carbohydrates. *N Engl J Med.* 2009; 360(9):859-873.

30. Redberg RF. Vitamin Supplements: More Cost Than Value. *Arch Intern Med.* 2011; 171(18):1634-1635.

31. McCormick DB. Vitamin/mineral supplements: of questionable benefit for the general population. *Nutrition Reviews.* 2010; 68(4):207-213.

32. Who Should Take Vitamin Supplements? *The Medical Letter.* 2011; 53(1379/1380):101-103.

33. Kris-Etherton PM, Lichtenstein AH, Howard BV, et al. Antioxidant Vitamin Supplements and Cardiovascular Disease. *Circulation.* 2004; 110:637-641.

34. Mursu J, Robien K, Harnack LJ, et al. Dietary Supplements and Mortality Rates in Older Women: The Iowa Women's Health Study. *Arch Int Med.* 2011; 171(18):1625-1633.

35. Drugs for Postmenopausal Osteoporosis. *Treatment Guidelines from The Medical Letter.* 2011; 9(111):67-74.

36. Do Calcium Supplements Increase the Risk of Myocardial Infarction? *The Medical Letter.* 2011; 53(1375):83.

37. Colon Cleansing. *The Medical Letter.* 2009;51(1312):39-40.

*Maclean, also author of *A River Runs Through It*, masterfully assesses our concepts of who we are in one of my favorite quotations: "The problem of self-identity is not just a problem for the young. It is a problem all the time. Perhaps the problem. It should haunt old age, and when it no longer does it should tell you that you are dead."

INDEX

About the Author

James L. Hardeman, MD has been practicing medicine for more than 30 years and has been living the principles of youth, longevity and good health for a lifetime. In addition to his demanding schedule of hospital-based medicine and a robust office practice, Dr. Hardeman has developed a variety of practical strategies for sustaining good health and a youthful appearance.

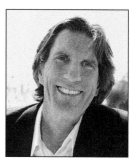

He is an honors graduate from the University of California at Irvine and Baylor College of Medicine. The recipient of numerous awards for patient care, Dr. Hardeman is Physician Adviser to the Clinical Nutrition Services at St. Jude Medical Center in Fullerton, California. Parents of two, he and his wife live and exercise in Southern California.

www.jameslhardeman.com